BEING BREAST AWARE

A Guide to Understanding the Breast and Breast Problems.

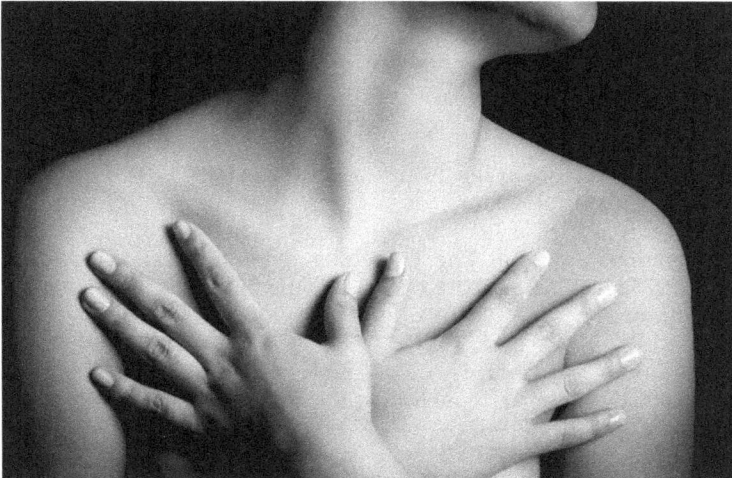

Dr. Shamanique Bodie-Williams

Being Breast Aware

A Guide to Understanding the Breast and Breast Problems.
A comprehensive guide on the breast for women including information on all lumps and bumps that can happen in the breast and
regular care for the breast.

TABLE OF CONTENTS

ACKNOWLEDGEMENTS

T o God who keeps me in His will and allows me the privilege of helping others, I give all glory, thanks, praise and honor.

To my husband Wellington Williams, thank you. I am continually blessed by you. You are indeed wise counsel at its best. Thank you for always being willing to listen to me.

To my daughter Lluvia, I LOVE YOU! Thank you for inspiring and motivating me to be the best that I can be. Happy Birthday now and for all your birthdays to come. I want you always trust God and live your best life!

To my and parents, Anita and Carlton Bodie – I give God thanks for you both daily. You always want the best for us and do your utmost to help us achieve our dreams. It is an honor to spend time with you.

Valdez, McCain and, Sharanna I love you and thank you for always encouraging me to continue to be me. Thank you for continually sharpening me. Thank you for being sources of encouragement and inspiration.

To Dr. Munroe, Dr. Chea and Dr. Francis– thank you for taking care of the many breast issues of women in believing the Bahamas over the years. Dr. Munroe thank you for taking the time to review my manuscript.

To my Wiley college professors especially Dr. Randriamahefa, Dr. Stuart and Mr. Fogg thank you for always believing in your students. Marshall, Texas - Wiley Wildcats! Dr. Lurain III thank you for my best memories as a fourth year medical student on your gynecology oncology service at Northwestern Feinberg School of Medicine.

To my colleagues in the Rand Memorial Hospital of Obstetrics and Gynecology Department, thank you. It is privilege and an honor to work with you - Dr. Pura, Dr. Espinoza, Dr. Miranda, Dr. Taylor, Dr. Issacs and Dr. Johnson - I thank you for your continuous support and hard work!

INTRODUCTION

B reasts are important; they have so many different purposes. Throughout history, they have been noted in science, art, politics, and religion. The functions of breasts are many: they can be used for your body image, to nurture children, to seduce, and to satisfy yourself and a partner. But they can also be a source of distress and pain, such as in cases where they may have abnormalities or disease. Breasts are complicated. In the following pages, I provide a simple guide for ladies who are trying to understand their breasts.

I speak from the point of view of a physician, a woman who has had breast concerns, and an educator. Being "breast aware" is essential. So, in the next few pages let me either confirm that you are breast aware, or encourage you to become more so. This guide has information to help you understand normal differences in the breasts, breast diseases, and procedures that may be done to the breasts. I want to demystify it all for you. While each of the topics you'll find here could easily have an entire book written about them, I want this guide to serve as a starting point of information and research. This book contains basic information about the breasts and breast care. My goal is to help a non-medical person understand and navigate the complexities of the breasts, including their anatomy, function, care, and the ability to assess them.

I will give you information to help you navigate the healthcare system. It helps to have options and to know where to go when seeking care. This book will also discuss some common (and not so common) non-cancerous issues that can occur in the breasts. We will discuss the risk factors for breast cancer and will briefly discuss it. However, this is not meant to be a breast cancer manual, as there are many resources available on that topic.

This information is meant to empower you, so that if you have a question about your breasts, you'll have direction on where you can go for answers. Feel free to make notes. Feel free to email me at bahamaswellnesscenter@gmail.com about topic areas that you would like to see included in future editions.

SECTION I
UNDERSTANDING THE BREAST

CHAPTER 1

WHAT IS A BREAST CONCERN AND WHO SHOULD I SEE?

❧

Song of Solomon 7:3 (New International Version) Your breasts are like two fawns, like twin fawns of a gazelle.

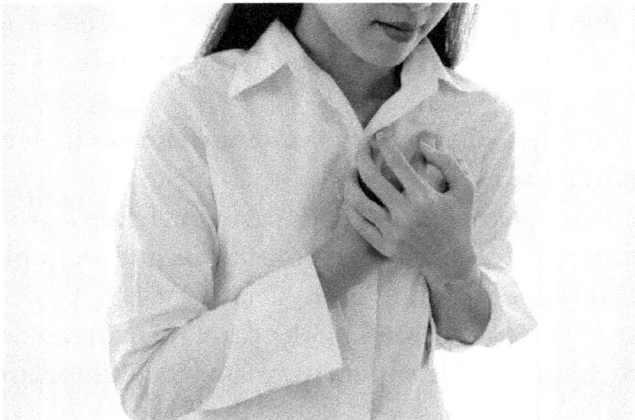

Figure 1 Woman with a Breast Concern

What is a Breast Concern?
There is a good chance that if you have breasts, at some point during your life, you may have a breast concern. A breast concern is anything about your breast that is bothering you or might seem like a problem to you or a healthcare provider. It may be related to the way that the breast looks, or it may be a new lump or bump that is discovered in the breast. The discovery may be made by you, your partner, or your health care provider. Having an issue that you are concerned about can be a source of uncertainty and anxiety for many ladies, and some gentleman. Information is key to helping you navigate the healthcare system and getting to where you need to be to get the appropriate help.

Who Should I See if I Have a Breast Concern?
The easiest and best person to see is a healthcare provider you trust. If you have a physician whom you trust and have an established relationship with, I recommend starting with that person.

If you are in the Western world, such as in the Bahamas, your gynecologist (female healthcare specialist) is usually the one who will evaluate you. In other countries, such as the United Kingdom, a general practitioner is often the person responsible for checking your breast health. Some problems, the gynecologist or general practitioner may be able to treat. For other issues, they may refer you to a general surgeon or a breast surgeon who specializes in breast care.

Below are the types of providers you may choose to see about your breast health:
Nurse Practitioners are licensed independent healthcare providers that can manage people's health conditions and help prevent disease under the supervision of a physician.

Physician's Assistants are healthcare providers who practice medicine under the supervision or in collaboration with a physician.

General practitioners are physicians who do not specialize in one particular area of medicine but provide general exams. They are the first point of contact with the healthcare system for many people.

Gynecologists are physicians that specialize in women's care. A gynecologist may be the primary care provider for many women.

Gynecologic Oncologists are physicians that specialize in women's care and have done additional training in the care of cancers in women, particularly endometrial, ovarian, and vaginal cancers.

General Surgeons are surgeons who have training that allow them to comfortably operate on most parts of the body, including the breasts.

Breast Surgeons are surgeons who have additional training in the treatment of breast diseases.

Internal Medicine Doctors, Endocrinologists, and Rheumatologists are physicians who have training in the management of chronic diseases, such as diabetes or autoimmune diseases. When a breast problem is related to a medical issue, you may be referred to one of these doctors for management or assistance with management.

Plastic Surgeons who specialize in breast reconstruction and augmentation can advise and perform any surgical changes that need to be made to the breasts.

If you do not have a healthcare provider, you can check with your insurance provider and ask for a list of covered specialists and then make an appointment. If you are not sure who to see, just go for an annual physical exam. You can mention your concern and the provider will give you advice on where to go.

Some hospitals and centers have specialized programs that are geared toward risk reduction and prevention of breast cancer. They specialize in providing services that are used to help screen, diagnose, and treat breast problems that may be cancerous or non-cancerous.

Summary Points

- There is a good chance that you may have a breast concern during your lifetime.
- There are different providers that you can elect to see for breast issues.
- If you have a breast concern, bring it the attention of a healthcare provider.
- You can factor in the cost of a visit prior to being seen by checking with your insurance provider. If you do not have insurance, you can ask for the out-of-pocket cost.

CHAPTER 2

MAKING THE MOST
OUT OF YOUR VISIT

❧

Jeremiah 33:6 (KJV)

*Behold, I will bring it health and cure, and
I will cure them, and will reveal unto them
the abundance of peace and truth.*

Congratulations, you have made the decision to seek help for your issue. Once you have made the decision about the healthcare provider you want to see, it is time to take the next step. Preparation is key to making the most out of your visit. Gather any records you may have from previous doctor visits. Take time to make a list of the following, including:

- Names of previous healthcare providers
- Medications that you are taking or have taken in the past
- Allergies that you have to medications or foods
- Family history of any medical issues

- Consultation notes or summaries
- Discharge summaries (if you have been admitted to a hospital)
- Test results from previous bloodwork
- Radiology reports, such as mammograms or ultrasounds

If you have any of the above documents, make a copy to carry to your visit. I suggest that you take the time to think about any medical problems in your family, including cancer. Think about who had what, and at what age. You may even consider writing them down so that you do not forget any details.

These details will be helpful to your provider in counselling you on your risk and how to approach screening you for breast issues and other non-breast related issues. Do not overlook anything. Your healthcare provider will decide if the information is important or not. If you have any medications that you are taking, including vitamin and herbal supplements, take them with you to the visit.

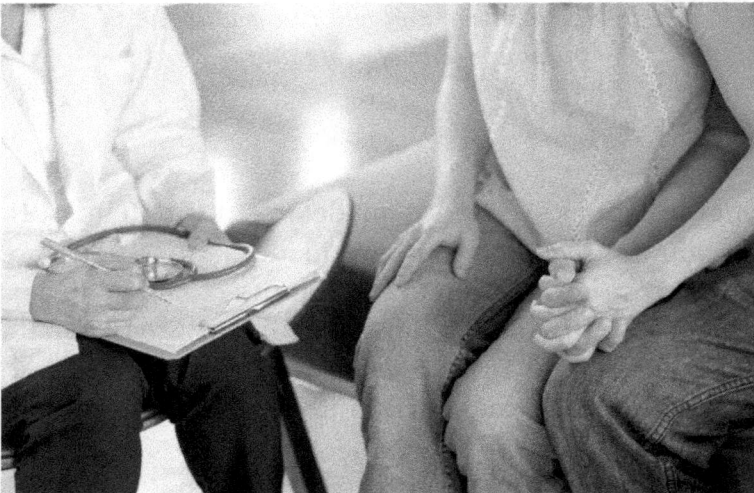

Figure 2 Female attending a doctor with a breast concern

Explain to the healthcare provider what your concern is. Once the healthcare provider understands the symptoms you are experiencing, they can help you. Symptoms such as pain, a lump, changes in the skin (such as thickening), or nipple discharge are important to pay attention to. Understanding your family history also gives the healthcare provider a chance to see if you are a candidate for genetic testing.

There are different parts of the visit that help the doctor get the information they need. These include the following:

- History of present illness (HPI)
- The physical exam
- Imaging

History of Present Illness
Addressing any problem including a breast problem includes taking a history from you. To obtain a history, the healthcare provider asks question about your complaint or concern. They may ask details about the issue, such as when the problem started, how long the problem has been going on, and what makes the problem better or worse. The provider takes the time to find out what is important to you. Once the history has been obtained, the clinician will usually perform a physical exam. The type of physical exam will depend on the clinical provider.

Physical Examination
The physical exam is when a healthcare provider (such as myself) inspects or touches different parts of your body to help us understand the problem that you are experiencing and determine a cause and possible treatment plan. The physical exam may or may not be limited to the breasts, depending on your concern and the physician that you are seeing.

Physical Examination of the Breasts

We have a variety of techniques to evaluate the breasts, but they usually involve similar steps, including inspection (looking) and palpation (touching). We are examining the breasts to find out if they are normal or if there is an abnormality.

Breast Inspection

This involves looking at the breasts. The provider may stand in front of you and look at the breast in two to four different positions, including:

- One or both arms at your side
- One or both arms over your head
- Hands pressed against hips with elbows extended laterally
- Arms over the head while you lie down

We are looking for symmetry (the similarity in appearance of each breast) and the nipple alignment (the way the nipple is positioned on each breast). We also look at the way the vessels (vein structures that carry blood away from the breast) are distributed across the breast. We are looking for any abnormality in the pattern of the blood vessels (abnormal venous pattern).

We also look at the color of the skin to identify any color that may appear abnormal, and we inspect the nipples for discharge.

Palpation

We ask the patient to lift one arm over their head while lying down and we palpate (feel) all four quadrants of the breast on that side. Here we are checking for size, shape, consistency, tenderness, and or nodularity. We also palpate the lymph nodes (areas responsible for removing infection) by the neck, and we may feel the lymph nodes under the arm.

Bloodwork and Imaging
Once the history and physical exam have been completed, the next step is to obtain any bloodwork and imaging that may help with assessment and planning for how to address the problem. (See section on imaging for more information.)

Economic Aspect of Care
If you have a problem, you should be seen by a professional and obtain medical advice about how to address it. If you ignore the issue and do not sort it out early, it could cost you (and your family) more distress in the long term. In short, it is better to tackle a problem early. If you are worried about cost, sit down and do a healthcare cost assessment. I suggest checking regularly to determine what your options are for accessing health care, in the event that you are faced with a medical problem. For the purposes of this book, we are examining care for the breasts. However, I suggest that you do an assessment of your options for all medical issues— particularly for preventative health maintenance—which is how you try to stop potential problems from actually happening.

Can I afford to go to the doctor?
This is a question that is important to face. When considering the cost, you have to take into account the provider costs, as well as the costs of the lab, imaging, and hospital fees for any procedures. Below is a breakdown of these costs.

Provider costs: If you have insurance, you can go in for your annual exam with your primary care physician or a women's health care provider. For example, if you live in the Bahamas, Caribbean, or the United States and see a gynecologist for your annual exam, they will likely do a breast exam as part of your physical examination.

If you have already done your annual exam for the year, you can also see the doctor about a specific problem. If you are using insurance, you can call or check online to see if your plan has a deductible (an amount that has to be paid before the insurance will kick in) or if you have a copay (a fee you are required to pay for a doctor's visit) or coinsurance (a percentage of the cost of a healthcare service that you will be required to pay). This information will determine the amount that you would pay to have a doctor's visit. Once you have a good idea of the cost in advance, you can try to set aside additional funds to cover the portion that would be your responsibility.

If you do not have insurance, you can check the out-of-pocket cost of the consultation, or look for a free clinic or government-sponsored clinic in your local area.

Lab fees, imaging and hospital fees: If your healthcare provider feels like you require bloodwork or imaging, you may need to check with your insurance prior to getting these services so that you can have an idea of how much it will cost. If you are paying cash for your services, it's also a good idea to check on the cost, as discounted fees may be available for cash-paying patients. Sometimes, specials or discounts may be available to you. For example, in the Bahamas, our imaging centers routinely offer discounts on mammograms in May and October.

How do I prepare financially if I do not have insurance? Being without insurance can cause a lot of anxiety. I recall feeling this way—even as a physician—when I first returned home and didn't have insurance for a few years because the cost was so high. It was something that I was not happy about, but I had a plan. For those that may be in this situation, I suggest the following:

- Consider trying to join a group insurance plan, as the premium may be less than an individual policy.
- Consider joining a catastrophic plan or one with a high deductible. This would give you coverage in the event of a large health care issue.

- Put some money into a health savings account. This amount will grow with time and may help to offset costs in an emergency.

Be aware of any free or subsidized healthcare services that are available in your community. Establish a relationship with a general provider —these visits are often cheaper than specialist care and you may be able to sort most problems out with this provider. If the issue is a complicated one, they would be able to refer you and help you access the public health system.

Summary Points

- Choose your provider.
- Make the most of your visit.
- Gather any past information that may help your doctor, such as medical records.
- Write out any medical problems, surgeries, allergies, medications you are taking, and your family history before you go to the doctor.
- Prepare a list of questions and concerns.
- Your healthcare provider will make note of your concerns and may perform a physical exam and order testing.
- Check with your insurance provider to find out if your visit is covered.
- If you have no insurance, find a local clinic or pay cash for your visit.

CHAPTER 3

NORMAL DEVELOPMENT, ANATOMY, AND PHYSIOLOGY OF THE BREASTS

❦

Ezekiel 16:7 (NIV)

*I made you grow like a plant of the field. You grew and
developed and entered puberty. Your breasts had formed
and your hair had grown, yet you were stark naked.*

Breast Development

Breast development starts when the embryo is about six weeks old.
The breasts start from two breast buds in the chest region, but they
do not fully develop in the womb. Their development continues
after birth—at puberty and then into young adulthood.

Breast buds are one of the first signs of puberty. When your
ovaries start to make hormones, the fat tissue in your breasts begins to increase. The growth of the breasts begins with the formation of secretory glands at the ends of the milk ducts. The breasts
and duct system continue to grow and mature with the development of many glands and lobules.

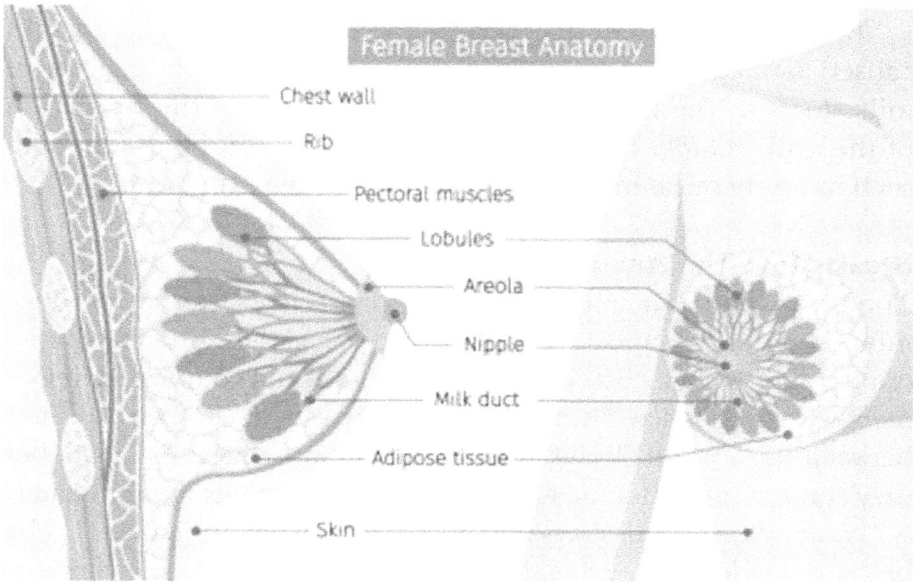

Figure 3 Breast Anatomy

The speed at which breasts grow is different for everyone, but the stages are the same. Breast development occurs in five stages:

Table 1

Staging of Breast Development	
Stage One:	In preadolescence, the breasts are flat and the tip of the nipple is raised.
Stage Two	Buds come, breast and nipple fat begin to form, and the dark areas of skin around the nipples (areola) get bigger.
Stage Three	Breasts are slightly larger with a different type of breast tissue (glandular breast tissue) present. Your breasts may be shaped like a cone first and then become rounder. The areola starts to darken.
Stage Four	The nipple and areola become raised and form a second mound above the rest of the breast.
Stage Five	Mature adult breasts are rounded, and only the nipple is raised.

Breast development may take 3-5 years. Each month, changes caused by hormones take place. Estrogen causes the growth of milk ducts in the breasts. Progesterone stimulates the formation of the milk glands. These hormones play a part in breast changes such as an increase in size, swelling, and tenderness.

Breast Make Up (Anatomy)
The breasts are also called mammary glands because they produce milk. Mammary glands are modified sweat glands (modified apocrine glands.) They start to develop in puberty and complete development with pregnancy. The mature adult breast is located on the chest between the 2nd and 6th ribs. The breasts are usually tear shaped, but they come in all different sizes. The average breast is approximately 5-7 centimeters in thickness and 10-12 centimeters in diameter. The breast is divided into two main regions, which include the main part of the breast (the circular body) and the axillary tail (tail of Spence). The average weight of the breast is 200-300 grams.

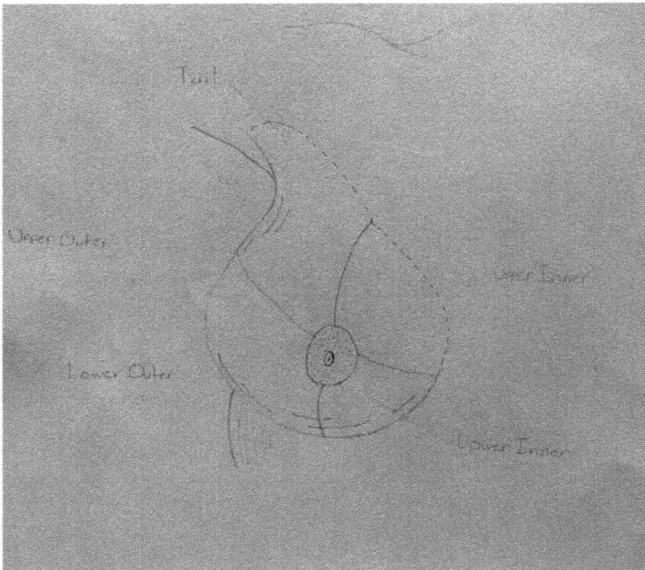

Figure 4 Right Breast Quadrants

The breasts can be divided into quadrants upper outer quadrant, the lower outer quadrant the lower inner quadrant, and the upper inner quadrant. Clinicians may use these terms to help describe the location of areas of concern in your breasts.

ANATOMY OF THE BREAST

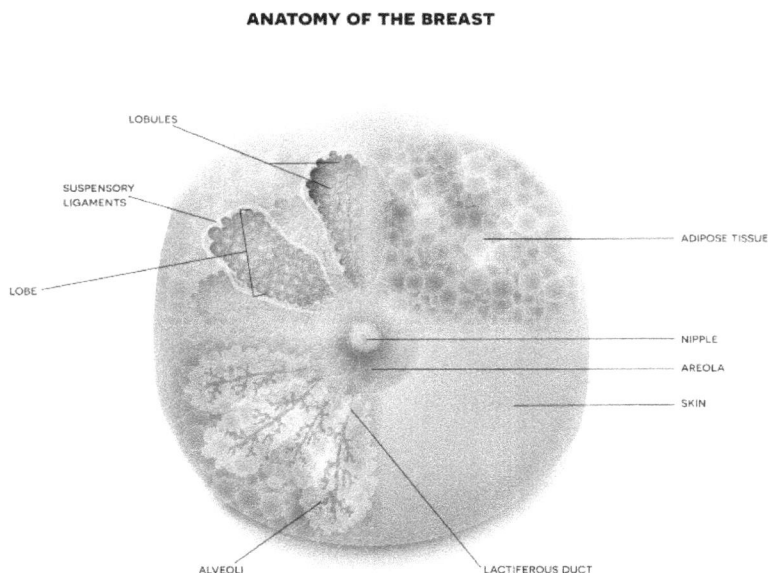

LOBULES

SUSPENSORY LIGAMENTS

LOBE

ADIPOSE TISSUE

NIPPLE

AREOLA

SKIN

ALVEOLI

LACTIFEROUS DUCT

Figure 5

The breast is made up the following parts:

- Skin: The outer most layer of the body.
- Nipples: The center part of the breast that is cone shaped and is surrounded by the areola. Nipples can be flat, protruding, inverted, or multiple. They have an average height of 10-12 millimeters and an average diameter of 11-13 millimeters.
- Areola: The colored area around each nipple. This may have different colors and sizes. The average diameter is 40 millimeters.

- Adipose tissue (Fat): This is the major part of the breast that gives it its size and consistency. Adipose tissue fills the spaces between the glandular tissue and fibrous tissue.
- Ducts: The tubes that transport milk into the nipple.
- Alveoli: The cavity sacs in the breasts that are the site of milk production.
- Lobe: These are triangle shaped.
- Lobule: These make up the lobes and look like clusters of grapes.
- Suspensory ligaments (connective tissue): This is supportive tissue made of collagen and elastic fibers.

Breasts are located on the front of the chest wall and usually go from the middle of the chest (sternum) to the middle of the underarm area (the mid-axillary line). They usually fall in front of the chest wall muscle (pectoralis muscles) and the tissue that holds the chest together (fascia).

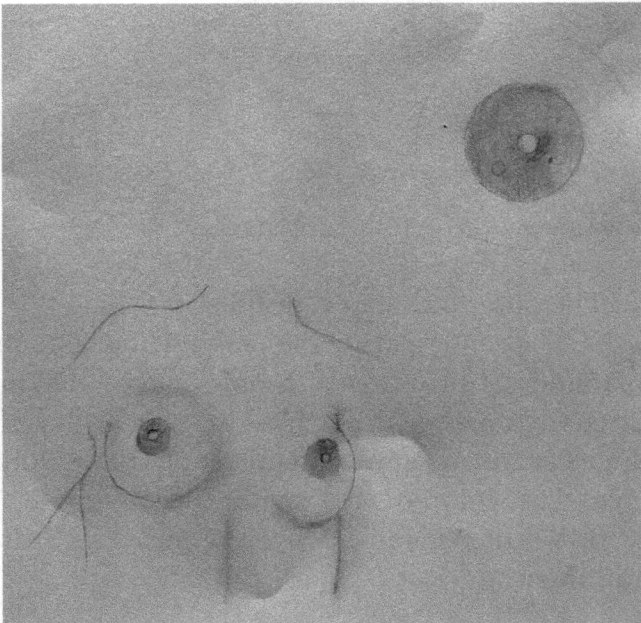

Figure 6 Breast and Nipple-Areolar Complex

The breasts are usually symmetrical (meaning that the left and right sides look similar), but they can vary or be different in size. One breast is composed of 15-20 lobes. Each lobe is made of 20-40 lobules. Each lobule has 10-100 alveoli. The alveoli come together to form a single duct that drains each lobe. Glands in the breast are called tubuloalveolar glands, which are modified sweat glands. The glands end in a lactiferous duct, which is 2-4 millimeters in diameter and opens into the nipple. Under the areola, each duct contains a lactiferous sinus where the milk accumulates. The myo-epithelial cells contract and help the breast secrete milk.

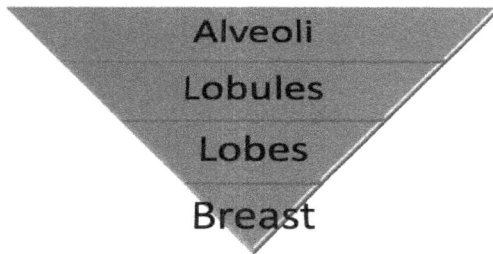

Figure 7 Pyramid Schematic of Breast Makeup

Breast Blood Supply
The breasts have blood vessels—called arteries and veins—that carry blood to and from them. They also have lymph nodes, which have many functions, including draining fluid away from them to help fight infection.

Blood flow to the breast is supplied by several different arteries. The superior thoracic, thoracoacromial, lateral thoracic, and subscapular arteries supply blood to the sides of the breasts. The internal thoracic artery (also known as the internal mammary artery) originates from the subclavian artery and supplies blood to the middle part of the breast.

The lateral part of the breast receives blood from four vessels:

- Lateral thoracic artery, which originates from the axillary artery.
- Thoracoacromial branches, which originate from the axillary artery.
- Lateral mammary branches, which originate from the posterior intercostal arteries (derived from the aorta). They supply the lateral aspect of the breast in the 2nd, 3rd, and 4th intercostal spaces.
- Mammary branch, which originates from the anterior intercostal artery.

The veins of the breast correspond with the arteries and drain into the axillary and internal thoracic veins. Veins are vessels that usually take blood away from a body part. The axillary vein and internal thoracic veins take blood away from the breast through the vena cava.

Nerves come from the later and anterior cutaneous branches of the 4th, 5th, and 6th intercoastal nerves. Different nerves play different roles in the body. For example, sensory nerves help the body feel things, while motor nerves help the muscles move. The breasts are supplied by branches of the intercostal nerves. These nerves are spread out throughout the breasts, and each breast has a different layout to the nerve supply. Another way to think of this is like two homes with different room layouts.

Lymph nodes are small bean shaped glands that are found all over the body, including in the neck and chest. Many of the lymph nodes in the breasts empty into the area under the arm (axilla). The job of lymph nodes is to clear fluid and waste and fight infection. The lymph nodes make a fluid that contains special cells, called lymphocytes, whose job is to eat bacteria or abnormal cells.

These lymph nodes also play a role in the spread of disease in the breast. There are three groups of lymph nodes that get lymph from breast tissue: the axillary nodes (75%), the parasternal nodes (20%), and the posterior intercostal nodes (5%). The skin of the breast also receives lymphatic drainage. The skin drains to the axillary, inferior deep cervical, and infraclavicular nodes. The nipple and areola drain into the subareolar lymphatic plexus.

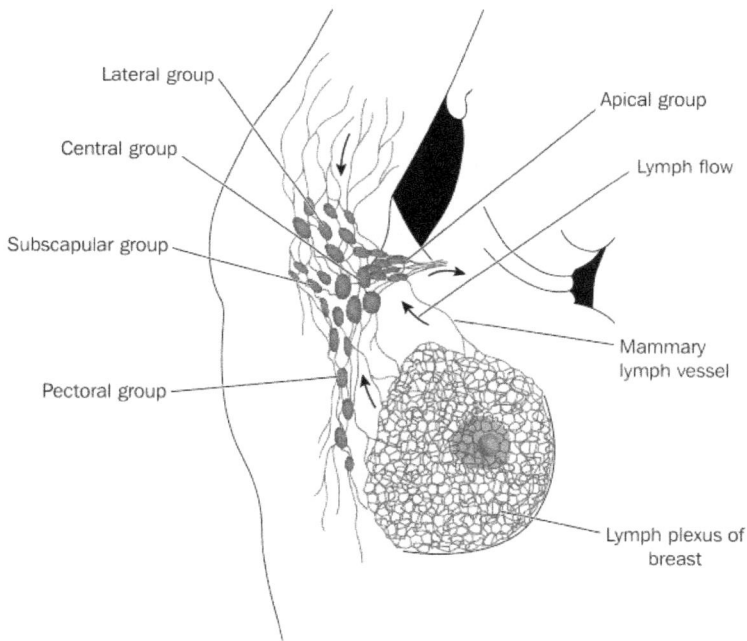

Figure 8 Breast Lymph Nodes

Appearance of the Breasts

The appearance of the breasts is different in every woman and is largely determined by your genetic makeup. There are some breast types which are more common than others, as discussed below.

BREAST SHAPES

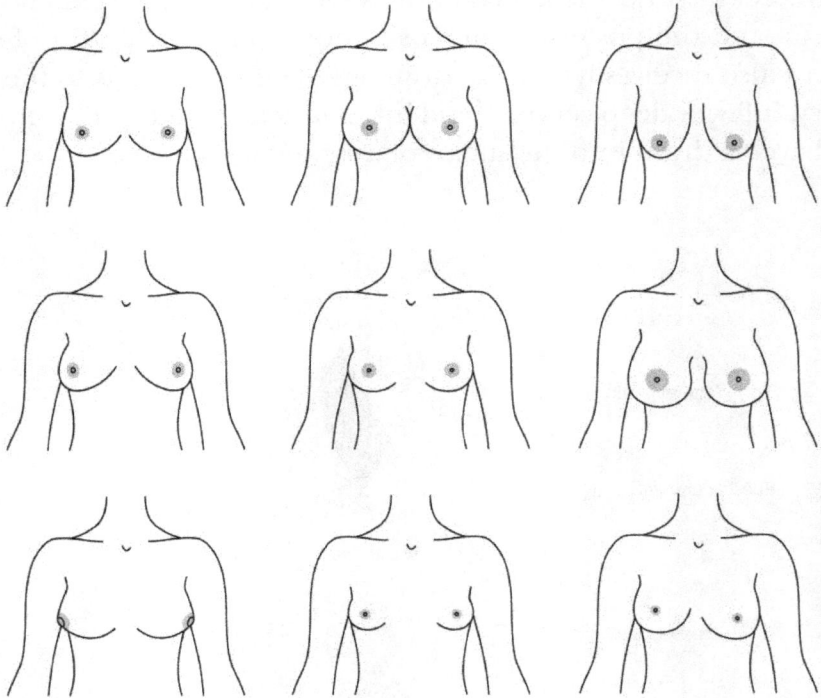

Figure 9

Standard/Archetypal

The "standard" or archetypal breast is round and full, with a small point at the nipple. This is considered the most common type of breast.

Asymmetrical

Many people have a difference in size between each breast. They can differ by a cup size or less and it is still considered normal.

Athletic
These breasts are more common in high performance athletes. They tend to have more muscle and less breast tissue and can appear wider.

Bell shaped
These are called bell shaped because they look like a bell, with a rounder bottom and a narrow top.

Close-set
Closet-set breasts sit more in the center of your chest and are very close together. There is very little space (or gap) between them. As a result, there's more space between you're underarm on the start of the breasts.

Conical
Conical breasts have the appearance of cones (e.g., orange traffic cones). This shape is more common in smaller breasts.

East West
The nipples on these breasts point away from the center of your body (outward). In other words, they point toward the east and west, hence the name.

Relaxed
In these breasts, the nipples point downward because the breast tissue is looser than in other breast types. You can think of someone relaxing or reclining—these breasts have a "laid back" appearance.

Round
Round breasts are circular shaped. They have an equal or even amount of fullness throughout the entire breast.

Side Set
Side-set breasts tend to be positioned more laterally (to the sides) on the chest wall. There may be a bigger space or gap in-between them and they may be further apart.

Slender
Slender breasts tend to be narrow and long with a tubular appearance and the nipples may point downward.

Teardrop
Teardrop breasts look like a teardrop. They appear more full at the bottom and less full at the top.

Appearance of Nipples
Like your breasts, your nipples are unique to you. They may contain different colors or features, that when combined, may make them look different. Below are some of the most common characteristics of nipples.

- The Montgomery glands may be easily seen, giving the nipples a bumpy appearance.
- Flat nipples are at the same level of the areola when they are not stimulated, but they can become erect with stimulation.
- Inverted nipples both nipples bend inward (see section on nipple inversion).
- Unilateral inverted nipples have one nipple that is everted and one that is inverted.
- Everted nipples look erect. They sit up and away from the areolae.
- Protruding nipples stand erect, further than everted nipples, even without stimulation.

- It is normal to have hair growing around your nipples. The amount of hair is different for each person and some people have more hair than others.
- Puffy nipples are when the areola and the nipple look like a pitcher's mound, which gives them a puffy appearance.

Summary Points

- Breasts start development in the womb and complete development with a pregnancy.
- There are five stages of breast development.
- The breasts have different parts.
- The breasts have a blood supply, venous supply, and lymphatic drainage.
- The breasts and nipples are unique to each person and have different appearances.

CHAPTER 4

THE BREASTS AND THE MENSTRUAL CYCLE

❧

Ezekiel 16:7 (NIV)

I made you grow like a plant of the field. You grew and developed and entered puberty. Your breasts had formed and your hair had grown, yet you were stark naked.

Changes happen in different areas of the female system at the same time. Throughout the menstrual cycle, some hormones go up and some go down. This affects the cycle, which is divided into parts. When talking about what takes place in the ovaries during your cycle, the terms used are *follicular phase*, *ovulatory phase*, and *luteal phase*. When talking about what takes place in the womb, the terms used are *menses*, *proliferative phase*, and *secretory phase*. The breasts respond to the different hormones throughout your cycle. To understand the breast changes that can take place, we will have to discuss the hormonal changes that are happening in the menstrual cycle.

26

The Hypothalamic-Pituitary Axis

The hypothalamus, pituitary gland, and the ovaries have an intimate relationship. The actions of one impact the other in what is referred to as the hypothalamic-pituitary axis. This causes hormonal changes that affect the reproductive endocrine phases, such as menstruation.

The Menstrual Cycle

Throughout the month, your body has different processes going on in the organs that play a role in the female reproductive system, which conclude in a period. The pathways are complicated, and they are referred to as phases.

- The follicular and luteal phases are based on what is happening in the ovaries.
- The proliferative and secretory phases are based on what is happening in the endometrium (lining) of the uterus.

Endometrium

Throughout the month, under the influence of hormones, this lining of the womb is thickening and preparing to maintain a pregnancy. Once the cycle ends and pregnancy does not take place, approximately two-thirds of the lining of the uterus leaves the body in the form of mostly blood and clots (period). Then the cycle starts over again.

Ovulation

Maturity of the oocytes (immature egg cells) happens in stages, just like your development happens in stages. Once you go through puberty, a few oocytes are recruited each month for further development, as a result of your hormones. Eventually one (sometimes two) will reach the final stages of development. These candidates are the ones that are released, which is called ovulation. The remainder then stop growing and disappear.

Breasts and the Menstrual Cycle
Breast tissue—such as the skin of the breast, the stroma, and the myoepithelial cells—all respond to the hormonal changes that happen throughout the month. The menstrual cycle is divided into the follicular and the luteal phase

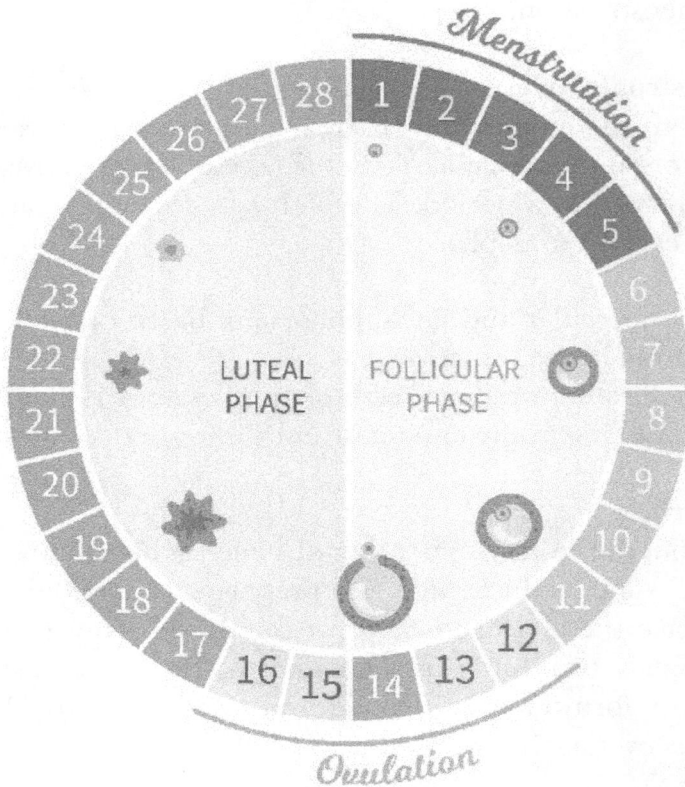

Figure 10 Schematic of Menstrual Cycle

Luteal Phase
The breasts may be tender and have an increased firmness and fullness during the luteal phase. The size of the breasts may also increase by 25 to 30 milliliters. During this time, there is an increase in blood flow to the breasts and water retention. The ducts increase in size and activity and the ductal system dilates. The

alveolar cells also change into secretory cells. In the time just before your period, the breasts may even appear to be more symmetrical than usual.

Follicular Phase
During this phase, the ducts system proliferates. The increase in estrogen improves the skin elasticity of the breasts and they get a "natural lift."

Menstruation
During menstruation, the cellular activity of the alveoli decreases. The ducts become smaller. The lobules increase in their amount and density. In other words, the breasts may feel lumpier than usual as the glands are preparing for a possible pregnancy. Do not panic. You can recheck your breast when your menstruation is over. Towards the end of the cycle, as the hormone levels reach their lowest, you may notice a decrease in the size of your breasts, and they may become softer than before.

Summary Points

- The menstrual cycle is divided into the follicular and luteal phases.
- The breast also goes through changes during a woman's monthly cycle.
- The breasts may have changes in shape, size, and texture throughout the month.

CHAPTER 5

SELF BREAST EXAM

❦

1 Corinthians 11:28 (KJV)

*But let a man examine himself, and so let him
eat of that bread, and drink of that cup.*

Breast self-exam has not been shown to decrease or increase the cancer detection rate, or the rate of detection of benign diseases. However, I firmly believe that the person who knows best what is going on with your body is you. You will be most likely to note if you feel something that is not quite right. We take the time to examine our face in the morning or evening. We tend to notice if there are new wrinkles or new moles. I am challenging you to take the time to give your breasts the same attention. In the previous chapter we discussed the steps a healthcare provider uses to check the breasts. In the following sections, we will review breast self-exam techniques.

Breast Self-Exam Techniques

Breast Self-Exam (BSE) is a good way to become familiar with your breasts. You can tell what is normal for you, and as you get to know your breasts, you'll notice any changes. You can do them yourself or you can have your partner perform the checks. BSE is also important for ladies who have had implants.

BREAST SELF EXAMINATION

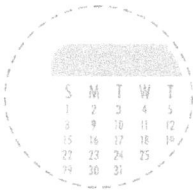

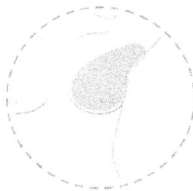

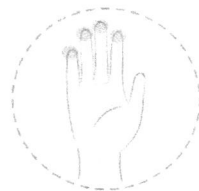

ONCE A MONTH,
2-3 DAYS AFTER PERIODS

EXAMINE BREAST AND ARMPIT
WITH RAISED ARM

USE FINGERPADS WITH
MASSAGE OIL OR SHOWER GEL

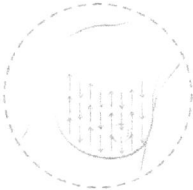

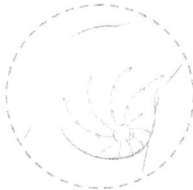

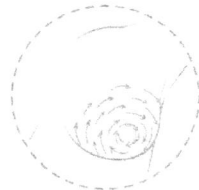

UP AND DOWN

WEDGES

CIRCLES

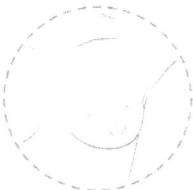

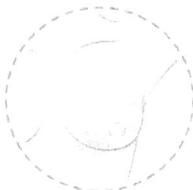

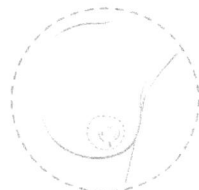

EXAMINE BREASTS IN THE MIRROR
FOR LUMPS OR SKIN DIMPLING...

...CHANGE IN SKIN COLOR
OR TEXTURE...

...NIPPLE DEFORMATION,
COLOR CHANGE OR LEAKS OF ANY FLUID

Figure 11 Techniques for Self-Breast Examination

If you find something during your self-exam that concerns you, bring it to the attention of your health care provider. I have had patients who discovered an abnormality in their breast that they found during a self-exam. I have also had patients who felt like something was not right with their breast, and breast experts nor imaging picked it up initially, but they ended up having breast cancer.

The best time to perform the exam is a few days after your period or, if you'll be taking hormone replacement therapy, the day that you start. When you examine your breasts around the same time each month, it makes it easier for you to keep up with. If you have gone through menopause, then you can check your breast at the same time each month.

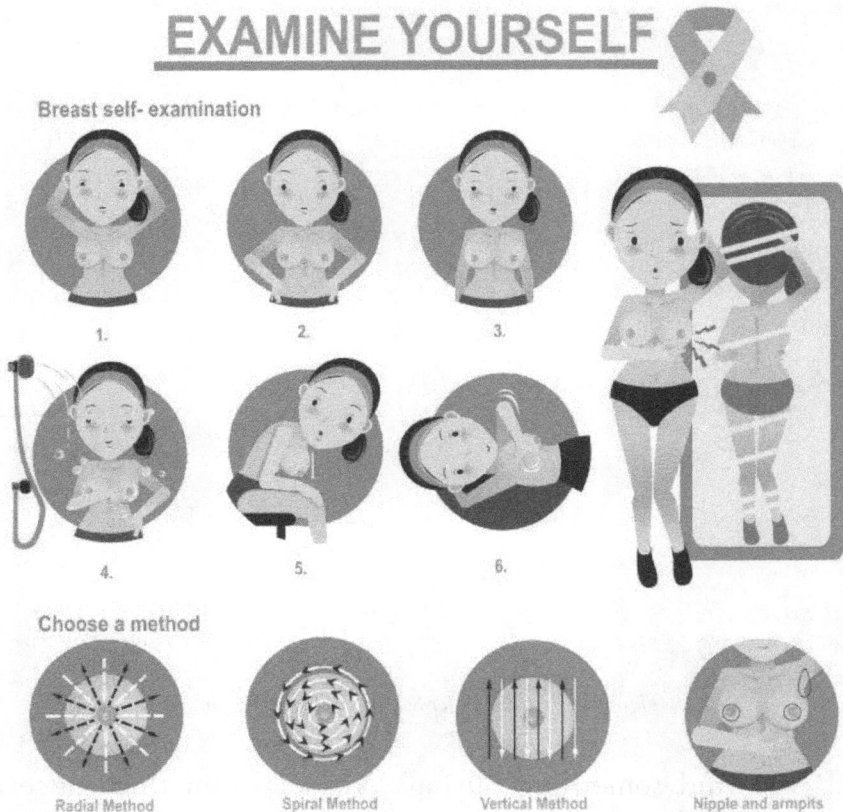

EXAMINE YOURSELF

Breast self- examination

1. 2. 3.

4. 5. 6.

Choose a method

Radial Method   Spiral Method   Vertical Method   Nipple and armpits

Figure 12 Alternative Positions and Methods for Self- Breast Examination

- Radial Method: Move in a radial fashion, simulating the hands of a clock.
- Spiral Method: Work in a circular fashion.
- Vertical Method: Start from the top and work to the bottom of each breast.
- Nipple and armpit: Check the nipple for any discharge. Check the armpit for any new lumps or bumps.

You can do your exam when you get out of the shower. You are doing almost the same exam that your doctor would do, but you are doing it yourself.

Stand in front of the mirror and look at both breasts. You are looking for anything that may be considered abnormal and checking for any of the changes that we discuss in earlier chapters, such as change in the skin color or redness.

Press your hands on your hips and lean toward the mirror. Then squeeze your shoulders back. You are looking to see if the breasts change shape in any way.

You can use the mirror to help you see the underside of the breasts. To do this, place your hands behind your head. Once you have completed your visual inspection, the next step is palpation. You can do this part any time, including during a shower or bath. First examine one side, then the other. For example, place your right hand on your right waist. Then use your left hand to check under the arm and the area above and below the collar bone. Once you have checked these areas, the next step is to check the body of the breast.

You can raise your arm up or place it behind your head. Use different levels or pressure (light, medium, and deep) exerted by your fingertips. You want to be sure to not miss any area of the breast. Do not lift your fingers completely off the breast during your exam to help ensure that no area is missed.

Summary Points

- Guidelines do not support breast self-exam for assistance in detection of malignancy, but I recommend you still do them to get to know your breasts.
- Breast self-exam allows you to get to know your body and notice any changes.
- Breast self-exam may allow you to find benign disease.
- There are different techniques that can be used for breast self-exams.

CHAPTER 6

BREAST DRESSING, SIZES AND FITTING EXPLAINED

❧

Song of Solomon 7:7 (NIV)

*Your stature is like that of the palm, and
your breasts like clusters of fruit.*

Breast Dressing
You may be self-conscious of the nipple showing through your clothes or you may need support. Some options would be:

- wearing a T-shirt or tank top under your clothes
- wearing a camisole (undershirt with thin straps)
- wearing nipple covers
- wearing bras: soft cup, underwire, padded, sports, or cropped top

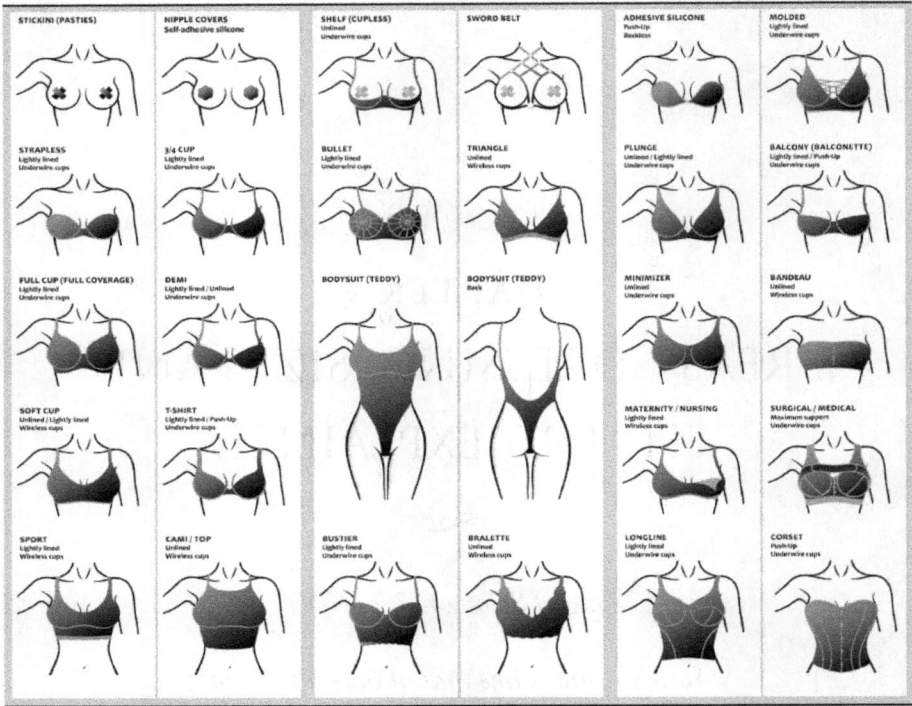

Figure 13 Different Types of Breast Dressings

Bras play several roles. For example, they can provide support for the breasts, they can also be used to make the wearer feel sexy and /or they can modify the appearance of the breast by making them appear larger or smaller. Bras have a long history that spans many years. Some ladies even choose to go without a bra. If you are a bra wearer, no matter the reason why you are choosing to wear a bra. you want to be as comfortable as possible. To be comfortable, you should select a bra that works for you. One step towards achieving this goal involves determining your bra size.

Determining Bra Size

To determine your bra size, you can:

- Estimate it
- Be fitted at a store (best option)
- Measure yourself

The bra size is made of the band number and a letter. For example, size 32 A.

To find out your band size, you would measure around your torso, just underneath your breasts. A 32 band size means that the measurement is 32 inches.

The letter refers to your cup (breast) size. It starts at AAA and goes up. To determine your cup size, you measure around the fullest part of your breasts. It should be parallel to the floor. Then subtract that measurement from the first measurement. The difference between the two measurements is your cup size. So, if you are 32 A, the measurement of the breasts would be 33 inches and under the breasts would be 32 inches. That gives a difference of 1 inch.

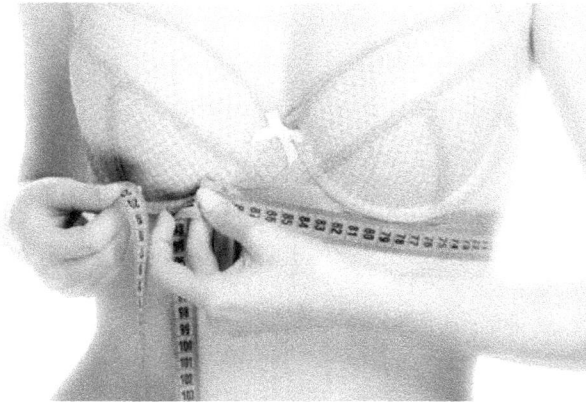

Figure 14 Self measurement of torso for band size

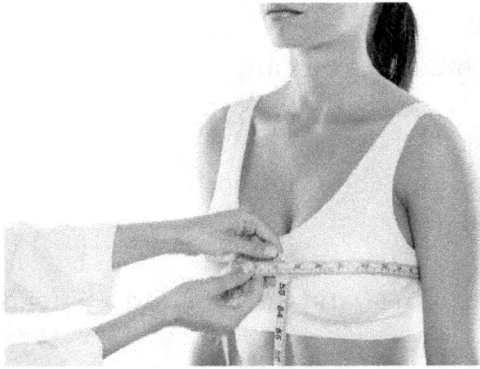

Figure 15 Measurement of the breasts by a third party

Table 2

Sizing Chart for the Bra	
Inches Different	Size
1	A
2	B
3	C
4	D
5	DD
6	DDD & F

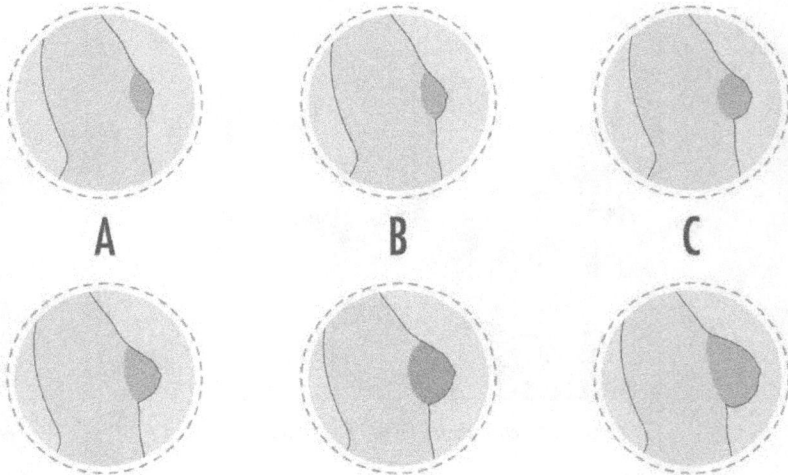

Figure 16 Schematic of Breast sizes

Finding the perfect fit of a bra may take a few tries. Your perfect fit will change as your breasts change. You may choose to go bra shopping by yourself but getting measured by a professional is helpful. Just like anything else the assistance of an expert is usually beneficial.

Make sure your bra is not too tight. You should be able to get a finger between the bra band and the body. With the cup part of the bra, you should not spill out the bra. If your breasts are coming up over the top of the bra, then you need to go up a size. If the band is riding up in the back or your breast are falling out the bra go down a band size.

Much of the support from the bra comes from the band. It make sure your bra offers you good support. Many bras look nice but do not give the support to the breasts that is needed. Breasts can be heavy. Good support will decrease the chance of having back pain. You also want to make sure the center part of the bra lies flat against your chest.

If you chose to wear a bra with an underwire – make sure it surrounds the breast without pinching any breast. The center gore of the bra should it should lay flat to the chest.

The right fit will allow you to be comfortable, contained, confident and in control of your day.

We might all have a bra that we love and do not want to get rid of, but bras do not last for forever. Some experts recommend that we change them after a year. The exact timing is up to you, but, once the bra has worn out, and is no longer supportive, it should be replaced.

"A good supporting bra can make your day!"
—*Dr. Pura.*

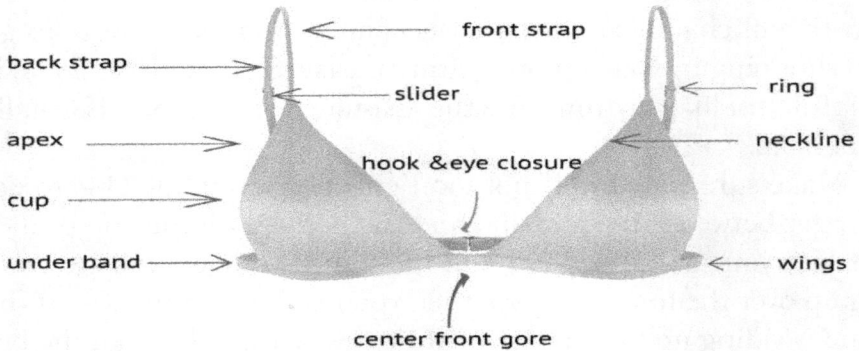

Figure 17 Anatomy of a bra

Summary Points

- Bras can be used to help your breast look the way you want them to look.
- Take the time to find out your bra size.
- Get professional help with sizing or someone else to measure you.
- Finding the right bra may take a few tries.
- Bras need to be replaced once the support wears out.

CHAPTER 7

BREAST IMAGING

❧

Imaging Used in Breast Evaluation

Imaging refers to the techniques (such as ultrasound) that we use to take pictures of what is happening on the inside of the breast. A picture usually adds information to the medical history that you have provided to your doctor, along with the knowledge gained from the exam. Below we will discuss various modalities that are used to evaluate the breast. Guidelines are changing, but the technology is also improving. Recommendations for breast imaging may vary by the group making the recommendation and the time. They often change as new information is obtained from scientific studies.

In the following paragraphs, we will discuss mammogram, ultrasound, and MRI. We use different types of imaging to determine whether what is happening in the breast is cancerous or not.

Indication for Breast Imaging
Your health care provider will determine whether they think breast imaging is necessary for you. Some of the organizations that provide information and guidelines on breast care and women's health have made the following recent recommendations:

American Congress of Obstetricians and Gynecologists (ACOG) Guidelines, January 2016. (Screening of Asymptomatic Women)

- Yearly mammogram at the age 40 and continue as long as patient is in good health.
- Clinical breast exam every 3 years in ladies ages 20-39.
- Breast self-exams are recommended, despite lack of clinical evidence.

The American Cancer Society (ACS) guidelines, 2015

- Women have the opportunity to begin annual screening between ages 40-44.
- Yearly mammogram for women with average risk starting at age 45.
- Annual mammogram for women ages 45-54.
- Starting at age 55, you should transition to every other year, but you can continue annually.
- Women should continue screening as long as their overall health is good and life expectancy is 10 years or longer.
- The ACS does not recommend clinical breast exam for breast cancer screening among average risk women.

US Preventative Task Force (Screening of Asymptomatic Women)

- Women may choose to begin biennial (every other year) screening between ages 40-49.
- Biennial screening is recommended for women ages 50-74.

Mammogram

There are three types of mammography:

- Conventional
- Digital
- 3D

Conventional Mammography

Traditional mammograms uses X-rays to make diagnostic images to evaluate the breasts.

Digital Mammography

Digital mammography uses a digital chip to record images of the breast, instead of traditional X-rays. Digital images enable you to have fewer total X-ray exposures and are less uncomfortable. The images of the breast can be viewed on a computer monitor or printed on a special film (like traditional mammograms). Digital images are particularly useful and better than conventional mammograms if you are younger than 50 or you have dense breasts.

3D Mammography

In traditional mammography, the details of the breast are viewed in one flat image. 3D mammography allows the breast to be viewed in a series of layers. The use of 3D mammography has been proven to significantly reduce false positives (seeing what appears to be an abnormality where there isn't one) and enables us to see small abnormal areas that may lead to detection of cancers at an earlier stage.

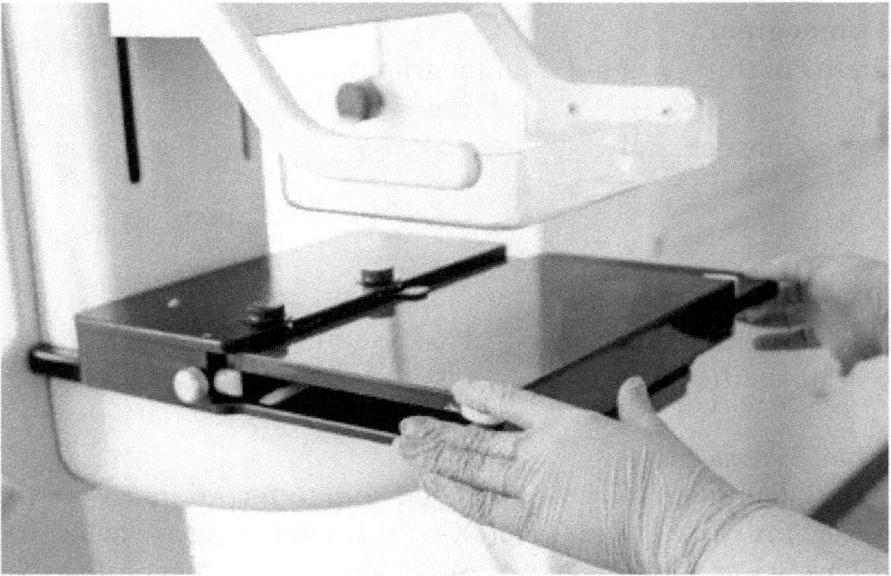

Figure 18 Picture of Mammogram Machine

This is a X Ray that is performed that looks at the breast from different points of view. the breast is compressed and looked at from the top and from the side. The images that are looked for include calcifications. There are different types of mammograms.

- Screening Mammography
- Diagnostic Mammogram

Screening Mammography

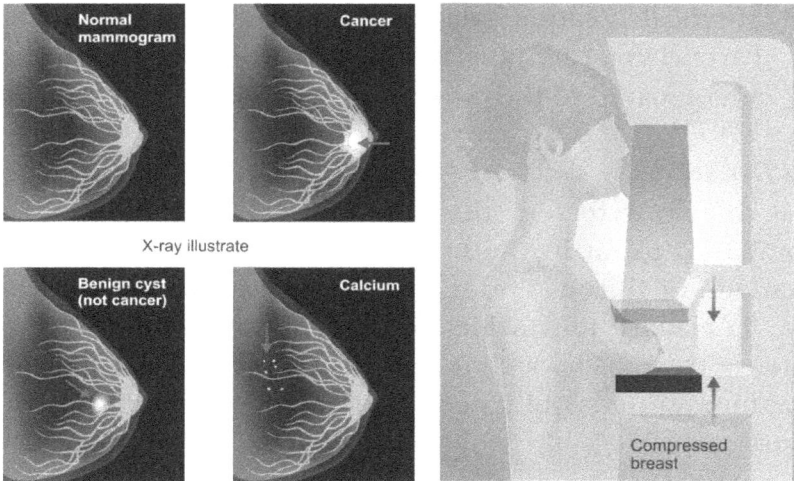

- In mammography, each breast is compressed horizontally.
- During a screening mammogram, the breast is placed between two plastic plates.
- The plates then are briefly compressed to flatten the breast tissue.
- Two views usually are taken of each breast.

Figure 19 Steps of Screening Mammogram

Diagnostic Mammogram

If your current or previous mammograms have shown areas of concern, you may be asked to do a diagnostic mammogram. This uses the same technology as a screening mammogram, but takes more pictures. The mammogram may also involve focusing on a specific area of the breast where they may take a magnified picture, called spot magnification.

Studies on X-ray mammography screening have been shown to improve survival, especially after the age of 50. Sometimes, we use mammograms and miss cancer. This is called a false negative, and can happen in 12-15% of cases.

The mammogram is used to look for:

- Density – normal non fatty tissue seen
- Microcalcification – discrete, scattered, fine, or course
- Parenchymal asymmetry – the grey white scale in one breast as compared to the other

Breast Density

Breast density refers to the amount of fibroglandular tissue as compared to fat in the breast. Dense breasts have a higher percentage of fibrous and glandular tissue, along with less fat tissue. There are four scales of determining whether a breast has dense tissue. The radiologist who is reviewing and reading the mammogram is obligated to comment on the density of the breasts.

Table 3 BI-RADS breast density

Type of designation	Description of Breast	Degree of fat vs. glandular tissue
Type I	Partially fatty	0 to 25% density
Type II	Somewhat or moderately fatty	25% to 50% density
Type III	Moderately or somewhat dense	50% to 75% density
Type IV	Very dense	75% to 100% density

Microcalcifications

There are also scales which look at the amount of microcalcifications. This is broken down into five types.

PROBABILITY OF DETECTING CANCER
IN DIFFERENT TYPES OF MICROCALCIFICATIONS

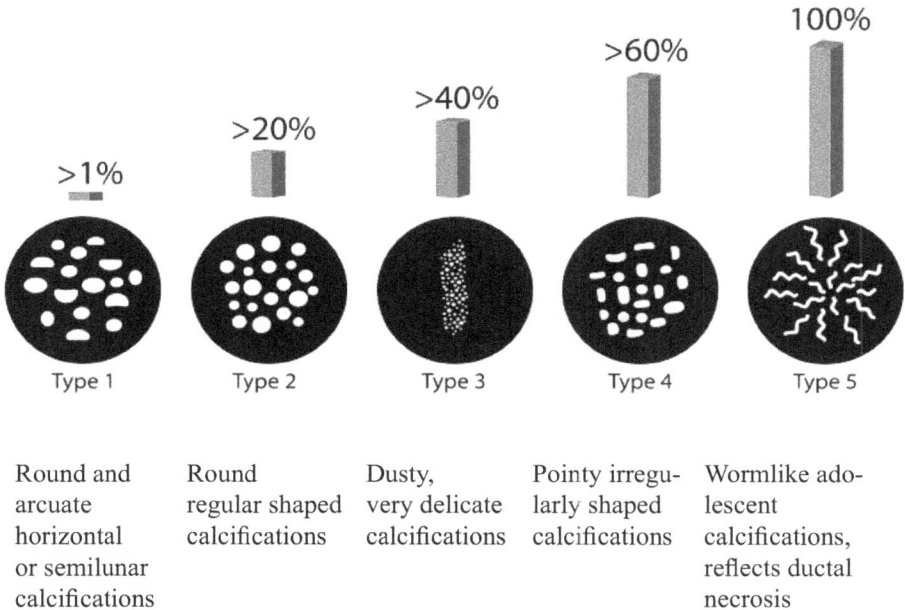

Type 1	Type 2	Type 3	Type 4	Type 5
>1%	>20%	>40%	>60%	100%
Round and arcuate horizontal or semilunar calcifications	Round regular shaped calcifications	Dusty, very delicate calcifications	Pointy irregularly shaped calcifications	Wormlike adolescent calcifications, reflects ductal necrosis

Figure 20 Types of Microcalcifications Seen on Mammogram

One of the disadvantages of mammograms is that it exposes the user to radiation, although it is important to note that the amount of radiation is small. In fact, a mammogram exposes you to less radiation than the amount you are exposed to in the world each year by going about your daily business (background radiation). Radiation exposure in radiology studies can be measured using the following terminology.

Table 4 Explanation of Radiation Measurements

Table 1. Some Measures of ionizing Radiation ⑩

Measure	Definition	Legacy Unit	SI* Unit
Exposure	Number of ions produced by X-ray or gamma radiation per kilogram of air	Roentgen (R)	2.58×10^{-4} C/kg
Dose	Amount of energy deposited per kilogram of tissue	Rad (rad)[†]	Gray (Gy)[†] 1,000 mGy = 1 Gy 1 Gy = 100 rad
Relative effective dose	Amount of energy deposited per kilogram of tissue normalized for biological effectiveness	Roentgen equivalent man (rem)	sievert (Sv) 1,000 mSv = 1 Sv 1 Sv = 100 rem

*International System of Units (SI) – these are preferred.
[†]For diagnostic X-rays, 1 rad = 1 rem, 1 Gy = 1 Sv.
Modified from Cunningham FG, Leveno KJ, Bloom SL, Spong CY, Dashe JS, Hoffman BL, et al. General considerations and maternal evaluation. In: Williams obstetrics. 24th ed. New York (NY): McGraw Hill Medical: 2014. p. 926–39.

The compression of the breasts during a mammogram can be uncomfortable. However, in my experience, I've found that the technician who is conducting the mammogram can make a difference in the amount of discomfort experienced.

The report from the mammogram will comment on the breasts and will typically make a comparison with previous mammograms the patient has had, along with a summary of the radiologist's thoughts. In the conclusion, the report will often have a Breast Imaging Reporting and Database System Scoring (BI-RADS) category.

BI-RADS

This is a scoring system used by radiologists (the person reading the mammogram) to help classify it for the health care provider, based on what is seen in the imaging.

Table 5 Breast Imaging Reporting and Database System Scoring

BI-RADS CATEGORY			
Score	Meaning	Action	Chance of Malignancy (percent)
0	Need additional imaging	Recall patient for additional imaging	Not applicable
1	Negative	Routine screening	Close to 0%
2	Benign	Routine screening	Close to 0%
3	Probably benign	Short interval follow up	>0% but ≤ 2%
4	Suspicious	Tissue diagnosis	4a. 2-10% 4b. 10-50% 4c. 50-95%
5	Highly suggestive of malignancy	Tissue diagnosis	>95%
6	Biopsy proven malignancy	Excision where clinically appropriate	100%

3D Mammogram Tomosynthesis (Digital Mammography)

This was developed in 2007. The X-ray machine rotates around the breast and takes multiple images at different angles. This type of imaging may be particularly helpful for people with dense breasts.

Breast Ultrasound

This technology uses sound waves and is not harmful to your body. The person performing the ultrasound may use gel and a machine to look at the breasts, including the skin, the underlying structure, and the breast tissue. Ultrasound may be used to evaluate a lesion to tell whether it is a cyst or a solid lesion. This test is often used in conjunction with mammogram to look at an area of concern. It is also beneficial in younger patients or patients with dense breasts. It is not usually recommended to be used as the sole screening test, as it may be more likely to miss cancerous lesions.

Molecular Breast Imaging (MBI)/Scintimammography/Breast-Specific Gamma Imaging (BGSI)
This molecular test is one that uses a radiotracer that is injected into a vein in your arm. The tracer then attaches to abnormal cells and a camera can then be used to locate the gamma radiation that is released by the tracer. This may be helpful when used in combination with mammogram in ladies who have dense breast tissue. It can also be helpful to assess a breast abnormality in ladies who may not be able to obtain a mammogram. The downsides of this type of imaging are that it exposes the entire body to radiation, it requires a radiotracer which some people may have an allergy to, it may not be able to detect all abnormalities or cancers, and it may need to be used in conjunction with other forms of imaging.

Magnetic Resonance Imaging (MRI) of the Breast
Breast MRI is usually recommended if you are considered high risk, such as having a lifetime risk of greater than 20%. These tests are good for differentiating between benign and malignant growths. They help determine margins and can see occult (hidden) tumors. This may help surgeons who are trying to determine which procedure to perform. Breast MRI may also be recommended if you have two or more family members who have had cancer, you have a history of chest wall radiation, your BRACA testing is positive, you have a genetic disease that increases your risk of cancer, you have dense breasts requiring biopsies, or if your breast assessment score shows that your lifetime breast cancer risk is increased.

MRI may also be used to help evaluate a breast lesion. The radiologist uses something called the Kaiser scoring system to evaluate lesions and assess the following characteristics:

* An enhancing lesion
* Breast MRI enhancement curves

- Margins
- Internal enhancement patterns
- Edema

Points are assigned for each of the five characteristics. If the points add up to more than four, a biopsy is recommended. It is not meant to replace clinical judgement, but it acts as a tool to assist radiologists in evaluating the image, thereby enhancing the recommendation (information) that they pass on to your clinician.

MRI Spectroscopy
This can be used in conjunction with MRI to more accurately diagnose a malignant lesion, as well as to monitor the treatment of breast cancer. It does have some limitations, such as cost, availability, and the time it takes to do the test.

Positron Emission Tomography (PET Scan)
PET scans are not recommended at this time for routine screening. This test is usually used to evaluate ladies who have previously been diagnosed and treated for breast cancer. It uses different radiotracers that are transported and then trapped in the cells as they carry out their day-to-day functions, such as metabolizing glucose. With many cancers, there is an increase in the uptake of glucose, so the radiotracer is more likely to be taken up into (and identify) abnormal tissue.

Positron Emission Tomography-CT Scan (PET-CT Scan)
This technique combines the strength of the two tests (PET scans and CT scans) to give information that is made of scanner images from both devices in the same session. This information can then be used for surgical planning and post-surgery treatment planning.

Positron Emission Tomography-MRI Scan (PET-MRI Scan)
Similarly, this technique combines the strength of PET scans and MRI scans to give information that is made of scanner images from both devices in the same session. This information can also be used for surgical planning and post-surgery treatment planning.

Alternative Screenings Methods
There are some other methods below that are used by some to evaluate the breasts. I strongly suggest that you discuss the use of these screenings with your health care provider before agreeing to one, as they can be unreliable and thus are not considered good screening tools. These include:

- Thermography
- Optical imaging tests
- Electrical impedance imaging
- Elastography

Thermography
Thermography is called thermal imagining. This test does not use radiation. Instead, it uses infrared technology to evaluate for temperature changes in body tissues. It is not thought to be sensitive enough to pick up cancer, so it is not recommended as a standard of care.

Optical Imaging Tests
This technology uses different types of light (without ionizing radiation) to take images of the breast tissue.

Electrical Impedance Imaging
This uses the electrical conductivity (electrochemical properties) of breast tissue to look for abnormal cells, which may be more likely to conduct electricity than normal cells.

Ultrasound Elastography

This technology uses ultrasound to evaluate the "stiffness" of a lesion. In other words, the ability of the lesion to change its shape when it is pressed with an ultrasound probe. The information gained from this test may help when deciding whether or not to have a lump biopsied.

Summary Points

- Different imaging methods are available to assess the breasts.
- Discuss your imaging needs with your health care provider.
- Screening is when a tool is used to check for any abnormality, before it becomes a bigger problem.
- Different organizations have different recommendations for screening.

SECTION II
BREAST PROBLEMS

CHAPTER 8

CONGENITAL OR ACQUIRED
BREAST DISORDERS

&

Song of Solomon 8:8 King James Version (KJV)

We have a little sister, and she hath no breasts:
what shall we do for our sister in the day
when she shall be spoken for?

Congenital or Acquired Breast Problems
Congenital problems are problems that we are born with. They are
structural or functional abnormalities that happened when your
body formed in the womb. Sometimes, you may not have any issues
with the difference. Sometimes, you may be uncomfortable with
it and want more information. When an issue happens as we get
older, we refer to it as acquired. Sometimes, we may identify the
trigger that caused it, such as a medication, illness, or exposure
to a particular substance, but many times we do not know the exact cause. Congenital or acquired abnormalities may be isolated

(occur by themselves) or they may be associated with other abnormalities, such as chest wall deformities.

Asymmetry of the Breast

The causes of asymmetry (when the size of one breast is different from the other) are not entirely known. This is usually not a cause for concern. Many women have a 10-20% difference in volume between each breast. The left breast may be bigger than the right, for example.

Nevertheless, if one breast seems bigger than the other (and your breasts have completed development), you can discuss it with your health care provider. If it bothers you, consider using padded bras or bra pads to even out their appearance. Many are able to deal with it without surgical intervention, but if that is recommended, you may be referred to a plastic surgeon. If you have no breast tissue at all, this could point to a health condition that may need to be treated so that your breasts can develop normally.

Accessory Breast Tissue

One to two out of 100 ladies will have an extra nipple or extra breast tissue. An extra nipple is called polythelia. An extra breast or breast tissue is called polymastia. Polymastia may look like a breast with a nipple and areola, or it may look like a lump under the skin, which is usually located below the normal breast tissue. If you have this, you may not notice any symptoms, or you may experience pain or discharge. This tissue can also develop noncancerous or cancerous lesions. If you have extra breast tissue, you may choose to have it removed. Your health care provider can advise you or refer you to a physician who would be able to remove it.

Hypoplasia (Macromastia)

Hypoplasia is when the breast tissue does not develop in a normal way during puberty. The breasts may be small and underdeveloped, and it can happen on one side or both sides. It may or may not be linked to other systemic illnesses. Treatment is usually done by a cosmetic or plastic surgeon through non-surgical and surgical methods.

Amastia (Absence of Breast Development)

Amastia is an absence of breast development, which is thought to be caused by the failure of an embryologic structure (called the milk line) to develop. It mostly occurs on one side of the body. Treatment for this disorder involves breast reconstruction.

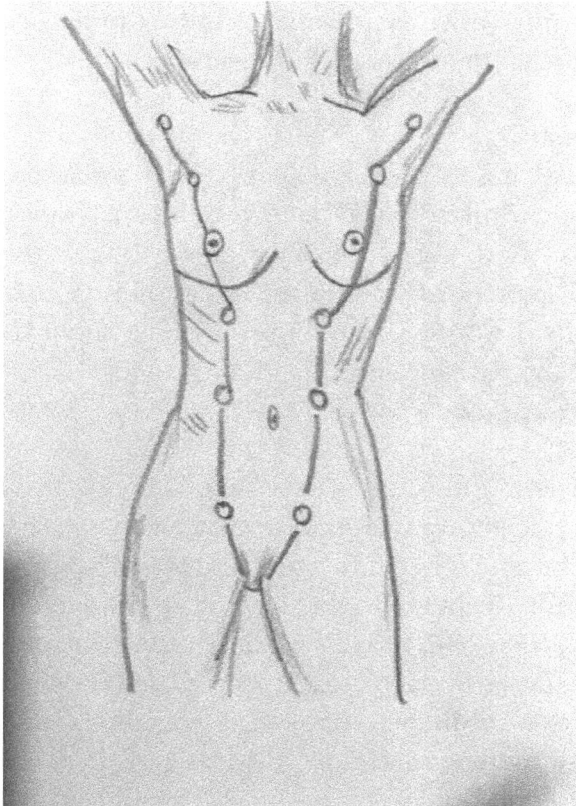

Figure 21 Schematic of Milk Line in Female (line runs from under arm to groin)

Amazia (Absence of Breast Tissue)

Amazia is a rare condition where the breast tissue is absent, but the nipple is present. This condition can be on one side or both sides. Some people are born with amazia, or it can be the result of trauma or radiation to the chest wall during childhood. Those who have amazia on both sides are unable to breastfeed.

Athelia (Absence of Nipple)

Athelia means that the nipple is not present on one or both breasts. Athelia is a rare condition that may be linked with diseases such as Poland syndrome, progeria (premature aging), ectodermal dysplasia, and Yunis-Varon syndrome. When Athelia occurs in both breasts, the breast tissue is usually absent as well.

Tubular Breasts

Tubular breasts have a sausage shape, with a narrow base and a trunk like appearance. This is caused by a constriction ring which has formed in the breasts and interferes with the way they grow. There are surgeons who specialize in correcting this defect with positive results. I would recommend seeking them out if you are considering having this condition treated.

Macromastia

Macromastia is a condition where one or both breasts increase in size at an accelerated rate. The exact cause is unknown, but typically the fat and/or glands will increase in size, which may be related to obesity or hormones. This change can occur over a prolonged period (e.g., 3-5 years) in adulthood or rapidly in adolescence. If the increase occurs around puberty, it is called virginal hypertrophy or juvenile hypertrophy. The sudden change in breast size may cause redness, itchiness, thinning of the breast skin, dilatation of the blood vessels, sagging, and possibly even break down (necrosis) of the breasts. The increased size of the breasts may also lead to neck pain and back pain, and may negatively impact one's body image. Medications have had limited (suboptimal) success in addressing this problem. Once the growth of the breasts has stabilized for a period of time, it can be addressed with plastic surgery.

Nipple inversion
Nipple inversion is when one or both nipples appear to point inward (as compared to pointing outward). This may be a normal variation in nipple type when a person is born with it. Other causes are inflammation and tumor infiltration. Inverted nipples may make it harder to breastfeed, but this can usually be addressed by manually pulling the nipple out or using devices that do so. Surgical procedures are also available that can permanently evert the nipple.

Summary Points

- Changes can happen in the nipple or breast tissue that result from how the breasts and nipples were formed prior to birth.
- If you are satisfied with the appearance of your breasts, no action needs to be taken.
- Your health care provider can make recommendations about treatment options if you are not satisfied with the appearance of your breasts.

CHAPTER 9

NON-CANCEROUS (BENIGN) BREAST LESIONS

❧

Psalm 103:2-5 (KJV)

Bless the Lord, O my soul, and forget not all his benefits:
Who forgiveth all thine iniquities; who healeth all thy
diseases; Who redeemeth thy life from destruction; who
crowneth thee with lovingkindness and tender mercies;
Who satisfieth thy mouth with good things; so that thy
youth is renewed like the eagle's.

This chapter will cover benign lesions of the breast. Benign breast disease is important to understand as it affects many women. Common breast concerns include a lump, pain, or discharge from the breast. It is thought that 1 in 2 women over age 20 will be impacted by benign breast disease at some point in their lives.

The good news is that most breast problems are noncancerous, but that doesn't mean that dealing with them is any less stressful or annoying. Having a breast lesion can cause a large amount of anxiety and distress as you go through the discovery, workup evaluation, and diagnosis phases. The benign lesions group accounts for the largest amount of breast concerns. It is thought that one million ladies are diagnosed with benign breast disease each year.

The symptoms that they present with and the type of problem tends to vary by age group.

Table 6

Differential diagnoses of benign breast changes classified by main symptom and incidence of breast cancer		
Symptom	**Benign causes**	**Incidence of breast cancer**
Pain (unilateral)	Cysts	2% to 7%
	Fibrocystic breast disease	
	Mastitis	
	Postoperative changes	
Palpable mass	Hyperplasia of the breast	8%
	Cysts	
	Fibrocystic breast disease	
	Fibroadenoma	
	Lipoma	
	Pseudoangiomatous stromal hyperplasia (PASH)	
	Hamartoma	
	Intramammary lymph nodes	
Nipple discharge	Hypothyroidism	5% to 21%
	Galactorrhea	
	Intraductal papilloma	
	Periductal mastitis	
	Ductal ectasia	

Causes of Benign Breast Masses

Variation of Normal Breast Tissue

Sometimes your breast tissue may be normal but can feel lumpy or have masses that feel abnormal. A biopsy may be required to determine that the tissue is normal, or your health care provider may decide to monitor the area.

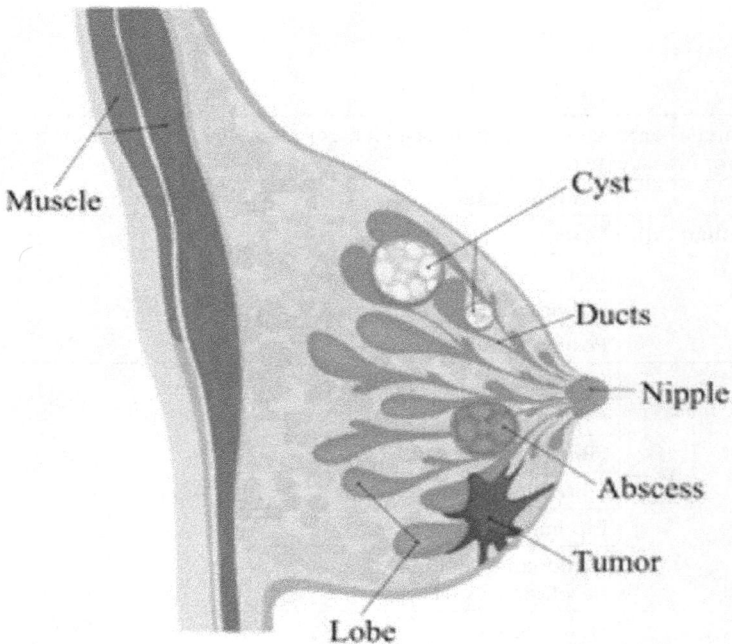

Figure 22 Benign Breast Disorders

Adenoma

Adenomatous lesions are benign tumors that grow from glandular parenchyma. The breast is made up of various glandular tissues, hence there can be of several types of adenomas. These tumors have different types and are characterized by the cells that make them up (e.g., tubular, lactating, apocrine). They can present in other locations of the body, such as under the arms, the chest wall, or the vulva. This problem may go away without surgery, or medication may be used to make it smaller. Adenomas are not thought to increase your breast cancer risk.

Fibroepithelial Breast Lesions
These breast lesions are made up of different types of tissue. They may be cancerous or noncancerous. They are broken down into the following types based on features of the tissue as seen under a microscope:

- Fibroadenoma
- Phyllodes tumor

Fibroadenoma
These are noncancerous firm lumps that may appear in the breast after puberty. They occur most commonly in the 15-35 year old age group and are the most common type of lump found in the breast. Fibroadenomas are the result of overgrowth of connective tissue (stroma) of the breast, which develops from the lobule. They have different classifications including simple, complex, and juvenile fibroadenoma.

This lump is usually firm and can be felt through the skin. The growth may be rapid initially, with an average size of 2-3 centimeters. You can usually move the lump around in the breast. It tends to occur on one side but can occur in both breasts. Many ladies do not have any symptoms aside from the lump. They are usually not painful but can sometimes feel tender, especially close to the time when you have your period. It is not fully understood what causes a fibroadenoma, but it is thought to be a sensitivity to estrogen.

Phyllodes tumor
Phyllodes tumors are rare breast tumors. They develop in the connective tissue (stroma) of the breast, in contrast to carcinomas,

which develop in the ducts or lobules. Although many are non-cancerous, some are malignant (cancerous). Treatment involves removal of the abnormal area, though sometimes additional treatment is required. These tumors tend to grow rapidly and can come back or recur when removed. Your oncologist can help you make decisions about treatment.

Fibrocystic Breast Changes
Fibrocystic changes are the most common benign changes in the breasts. This condition is noncancerous and is affected by your hormones. As the hormone levels change, the epithelial cells increase, and the ducts widen. Fibrocystic breasts may have cysts or an increase in the connective tissue (fibrosis) which may be felt on examination.

Fibrocystic breast changes can happen in one or both breasts. They can be extremely painful, especially around menses or the time of ovulation. Around this time, the breasts may feel especially lumpy, but this may improve once the period starts. Pain medication, vitamins, and decreasing caffeine intake may help reduce the pain. In some cases, birth control pills may also be used to help manage the pain.

Breast Cysts
A cyst is a sac filled with fluid. These can occur anywhere in the body, including the breasts. Cysts are common and are most frequently found in the 40-50 year old age group. They may feel round and spongy and can occur on one or both sides. Cysts may increase before your period and go away afterward. Sometimes, they are large, tender, and cause pain. If this is the case, a health care provider may empty the cyst of its contents by a procedure called fine needle aspiration (see section on Procedures in the Breast) and send the fluid for additional testing. The fluid that is taken out may have different colors or vary in color.

Breast cysts are categorized as either simple or complex, depending on how they appear on an ultrasound. Complex cysts have an increased risk of cancer. The doctor may send the fluid that has been taken out of the cyst to the laboratory so that it can be examined under a microscope. Once the cyst has been drained, the health care provider will recheck the area to see if additional testing and procedures are needed.

Breast Epidermal Inclusion Cyst (Epidermoid or Sebaceous Cyst)
The epidermal inclusion cyst is a benign breast lesion. These cysts are usually found in the skin or subcutaneous tissue. They are most likely to be found in the inframammary fold and are usually well-circumscribed, rounded, soft-tissue density lesions, close to the skin surface. They may appear small and can often be identified via ultrasound. Some problems encountered with these include infection, inflammation, cyst rupture causing a foreign-body or granulomatous reaction, abscess formation, or malignant transformation into a low-grade squamous cell carcinoma.

Sclerosis of the Breast
Sclerosis of the breast, or a sclerosing lesion of the breast, is a benign area of hardened breast tissue. The most common types of these lesions are radial scar/complex sclerosing lesions and sclerosing adenosis. Although this occurs most commonly in women in their 30s to 40s, it can happen at any age. Sclerosing adenosis may occur as you age and is the result of tissue growth in the breast lobules.

If you have this condition, you may not have any symptoms, or you may have a small lump, usually under 1 centimeter in size. Some may have pain in their breast, but this is rare. Sclerosing adenosis can be diagnosed through mammogram. If it is suspected that you have sclerosing adenosis, a biopsy (sampling of the tissue) may be needed to make a definite diagnosis.

If an excision biopsy is needed to remove the affected area, the tissue is sent to a laboratory where it is looked at under a microscope to confirm the diagnosis. Once the diagnosis has been confirmed, no further treatment is needed. This does not increase your risk of developing breast cancer.

Radial scars and complex sclerosing lesions are also benign areas of hardened breast tissue. They are similar to sclerosing adenosis, but are usually larger than 1 centimeter in size. The name describes how the area looks in imaging. Most people will not notice any symptoms, and these are often only found during a routine mammogram.

Your health care provider may suggest that you have the tissue sampled or removed to confirm the diagnosis because radial scars and complex sclerosing lesions may look similar to breast cancer on a mammogram. The removed breast tissue will be sent to a laboratory for examination. To date, it is not clear whether a radial scar or complex sclerosing lesion might slightly increase your risk of breast cancer. Your health care provider would review the current guidelines and make appropriate recommendations to you.

Galactocele

This is a cyst that is filled with milk and is a result of milk retention. This occurs due to a plugging of the lactiferous duct. If this happens, you may feel a firm lump in the breast. This may happen if you are breastfeeding or if you have recently completed lactation. A galactocele is one of the most common tumors found in the postpartum period. These tumors can be hard to distinguish from cancer, so sometimes additional imaging is required. Once your clinician is comfortable that it is milk, they may recommend draining it. This may help with the diagnosis and also alleviate any discomfort from the cyst. A galactocele does not increase your risk of breast cancer.

Fatty Tissue Tumors

Fat Necrosis

This is an inflammatory condition that usually comes after trauma to the breast which occurred weeks or months before. The trauma to the breast causes cell death, resulting in a lump of dead tissue in the breast. You may not remember the trauma to the breast and the area may even be painless. There are two types of necrosis—one looks like cancer and the other has the appearance of a cyst. The latter is called an oil cyst (the fat cells release their contents thereby forming a cyst). It may be difficult to distinguish the appearance of fat necrosis and malignancy; therefore, some researchers recommend biopsy. If the area is tender and soft, your doctor may be able to sample the area. This is not associated with an increased risk of cancer.

Lipoma

This a non-cancerous lump in the breast that is made of fat cells and is surrounded by a thin capsule. The tumor is usually a non-tender lump. If it is greater than 10 centimeters in diameter, it is considered a giant lipoma. Mammogram and ultrasound may miss this lump and may not be helpful in making a diagnosis, so this is usually diagnosed during a clinical exam. A lipoma can cause the breasts to be asymmetric, or increased in size on one side. If you have a lump that is increasing in size quickly, or your health care provider is not sure, they may suggest that this be removed.

Other Types of Breast Lesions

Hamartoma

A hamartoma is a rare, smooth, painless lump formed by the overgrowth of mature breast cells. These lesions may have different amounts of fatty, fibrous, or smooth muscle tissue, and/or gland tissue. This type of lesion is rarely associated with cancer. The treatment is usually excision (removal) of the area of concern. This allows the tissue to be sent to the pathologist for review so that a diagnosis can be obtained or confirmed.

Hematoma
This is when there is an area that has a collection of blood from internal bleeding. This can be a result of trauma or surgery. If the hematoma is small, it will often resolve without any additional intervention. If the hematoma is large, it may require drainage to assist with the pain and to expedite the healing process.

Granular Cell Tumor (GrCT) of the Breast
This is a rare, often benign tumor, which is possibly of neural origin (Schwann cell origin). These occur most frequently in premenopausal women. They usually present with a hard, palpable mass in the inner quadrant of the breast, which may clinically be similar to how a malignancy would present.

Neuroma
This tumor is an overgrowth of nerve cells. It can happen as a result of trauma via breast surgery to treat cancer or a cosmetic procedure. A neuroma is nonneoplastic reactive proliferation of the proximal end of a partially transected or severed nerve. The disorganized tangled mass of nerve cells is a result of a failed attempt to regenerate in a useful way. This neuroma may produce severe refractory nerve pain, functional impairment, and disrupt your quality of life.

Neurofibroma
A neurofibroma is a lesion that involves nerves or the covering of nerves. When this happens in the breast it is called a breast

schwannoma or breast neurofibroma. They can develop from a single or multiple nerve endings. These are most likely non-cancerous, but some types do have a chance of becoming cancerous. These lesions can be lumps that may be itchy or painful since they are related to nerves. The treatment of these lumps usually involves removing them through surgery. Although they can develop sporadically, they are usually linked with genetic disorders called neurofibromatosis (NF). Breast neurofibromas are generally associated with NF type 1, while breast schwannomas are associated with NF type 2.

1. **Neurofibromatosis Type1** (NF1) is a disorder that may result in formation of multiple neurofibromas and spots of increased or decreased skin pigmentation (cafe-au-lait spots).
2. **Neurofibromatosis type 2** (NF2) is a disorder that may cause tumors in the brain or spinal cord.

Tumors of the Nipple
Tumors of the nipple include:

- Nipple adenoma
- Infiltrating syringomatous adenoma

A nipple adenoma is an overgrowth in the lactiferous ducts of the nipple that causes a palpable nodule in the nipple. The nipple may have an ulcer or discharge. The treatment is to excise (remove) the adenoma. One must also be aware that sometimes the nipple adenoma can co-exist with breast cancer in the same or opposite breast.

Infiltrating syringomatous adenoma tend to affect one breast (unilateral). It usually presents as a firm mass that is in the areola region. The lesion may cause the nipple to be itchy, have discharge, or be inverted. The treatment is surgical removal, but they may re-occur if they are not completely removed.

Summary Points

- If you notice a lump in your breast, bring it to the attention of your health care provider.
- Your health care provider uses your patient history and clinical exam to make the diagnosis. They may confirm the findings with an ultrasound.
- Tumors may occur in the breast or the nipple-areolar complex.
- Benign tumors may be treated with surgical excision.

CHAPTER 10

INFECTIONS IN THE BREAST

❧

Exodus 23:25 (KJV)

And ye shall serve the Lord your God, and he
shall bless thy bread, and thy water; and
I will take sickness away from the midst of thee.

Inflammation in the Breast

Inflammation in the breast can be caused by bacteria (infection) or it can be caused by other things that are nonbacterial, such as fungus. Other conditions, such as lupus, can also cause inflammation in the breast. These conditions may cause the breast to become red, irritated, inflamed, and painful. You may also have an area of the breast that becomes hardened, and some may experience nipple discharge. Inflammation of the breast is referred to as mastitis.

MASTITIS

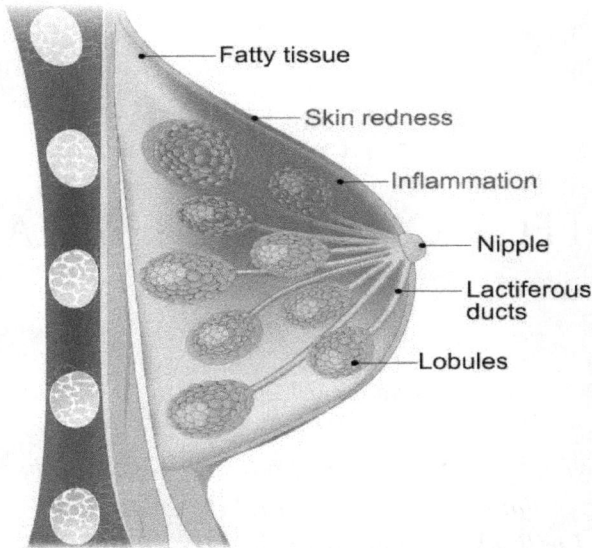

Figure 23 Breast Tissue Response to Mastitis

Mammary Duct Ectasia (Periductal Mastitis)

Mammary duct ectasia can happen at any age, but is most common in ladies who are approaching menopause. A blockage in the subareolar ducts may cause the duct to shorten and widen. As a result, you may have nipple discharge, which may be sticky and appear different colors. The breast discharge will usually stop on its own. If it does not, your health care provider may refer you to a surgeon to remove the problem area. This does not increase your risk of cancer.

Mondor's disease

Mondor's disease (superficial thrombophlebitis) is a rare and benign (noncancerous) condition that can occur in both women and men, but is more commonly found in women. It is caused by inflammation of a vein in the breast or chest wall, which makes the vein visible under the skin. Although Mondor's disease can affect any of the veins in the breast, it usually affects those on the outer side of the breast or under the nipple. Although Mondor's disease does not cause breast cancer, nor does it increase the risk of breast cancer, on very rare occasions it can be a sign that there is cancer in the breast.

Risk factors for Mondor's disease include:

- Breast biopsy, surgery, or reconstruction
- An injury to the breast
- Wearing a very tight bra
- Vigorous exercise

Mondor's disease looks like a long narrow cord under the skin, which is often red and painful to touch. Over time, the narrow cord becomes a painless, tough band where the skin becomes pulled in. You may also notice a shallow groove that is seen over the cord when the arm on the affected side is raised. This causes the skin over the breast to stretch, which makes the cord, easier to notice.

If you suspect you have Mondor's disease, your health care provider will examine your breasts and may also ask you to have a mammogram and ultrasound to help make the diagnosis. Mondor's disease will usually improve with time. Although the pain may resolve after a few of weeks, the cord can remain for a longer time period, such as a few months.

If you have Mondor's disease, you may need to use a pain reliever, such as an anti-inflammatory medication that you'll take orally or apply to the affected area. A warm compress or green cabbage leaves may also be helpful. Resting the arm and wearing a well-fitting bra may help with improving discomfort as well.

Mastitis and Breast Abscesses

Mastitis and breast abscesses are infections in the breast that are mostly caused by common bacteria, such as *Staphylococcus aureus*, or A *Streptococcus*, or *Enterococcus*. The affected breast may be tender, red, and warm. You made be sent to do lab work, such as a complete blood count or blood cultures (if you have fever). Your health care provider may ask you to get an ultrasound of the breast. Mastitis and breast abscesses are usually treated with a course of antibiotics. An abscess is a collection of pus (liquid produced by infected tissue, often appearing yellow or green) that has accumulated in the body. In the case of an abscess, the area may need to be opened and drained (incision and drainage) in order to decrease the amount of infection.

Tuberculosis and the Breasts

Tuberculosis is caused by *Mycobacterium tuberculosis* and it accounts for a small number of breast lesions. This is a single lump found in the in middle or outer part of the breast. Aside from the lump, you may not have any symptoms. However, a small number of patients may experience fever, fatigue, and night sweats. Risk factors for tuberculosis include if you are breastfeeding, had trauma to the breast, have AIDS, or have an infection in the breast. This lesion in the breast can be difficult to tell from other breast issues.

There are different forms of breast tuberculosis, including:

1. Nodular form
2. Diffuse or disseminated form
3. Sclerosing form
4. Tuberculosis mastitis obliterna
5. Acute miliary tuberculosis

The infection happens when you are exposed to the bacterium or you have breaks in the nipple.

It may spread to nearby areas, such as the ribs, the lungs, or the abdomen. The way that we assess for it includes trying to take a culture of the breast, but the bacteria is only found in a small number of cases. Health care providers may also try to take out the entire affected area. Fine needle aspiration can also be used to help with diagnosis. (See section on Fine Needle Aspiration.)

Medications can be used to treat these breast lesions. Most cases are successfully treated when the correct medication is used. Because this infection is rare, your health care provider has to have a high level of suspicion to go forward with this route of treatment.

Granulomatous Mastitis
This a benign disorder of the breast that may mimic cancerous conditions of the breast. The cause is not yet known but is thought to have to do with an autoimmune response. It is also thought to be linked to a bacterium called *Corynebacterium spp.*

Granulomatous mastitis can appear after pregnancy. You may notice tenderness, or you may not have any symptoms. This is not related to breastfeeding and may be caused by a reaction to the oral contraceptive pill. The condition may cause a hard mass between 1-8 centimeters, which may be found anywhere in the breast but may not affect the area next to the areola.

Actinomyces
This is a bacterium that is found in the gastrointestinal system and the female genital tract. If the protective system of the breast is disrupted, this can serve as an entry way to the breast. This infection usually causes breast abscesses that are chronic and may come and go. It is difficult to distinguish actinomyces from cancer.

Non-Bacterial Infections

Worm and Parasitic Infections
Some types of worms and parasites can infect the breasts. These infections may be more common in subtropical climates. They can cause a firm mass in the breast and are usually diagnosed with fine needle aspiration. When diagnosing, the provider may be able to see the parasite and/or the cells that result from the inflammation caused by the worm or parasite in the tissue may be noted. These worm and parasitic infections are treated with medications that kill or weaken them so that your body is able to dispose of them. Some of the most common types of these infections are:

- Filariasis
- Myiasis
- Cysticercosis
- Schistosomiasis

Filariasis
Lymphatic filariasis is caused by nematodes (parasitic worms) that live in the lymphatic vessels and lymph nodes of a human host. These worms are transmitted to a human through the bite of a mosquito. *Wuchereria bancrofti* is the type of parasitic worm that is the most common cause of infections in humans. Although the inguinal lymph nodes and lower extremities are most commonly involved in this infection, the breasts and genitalia can also be affected. The microfilaria can get into the lymphatic vessels of the mammary gland and develop into adult worms, affecting lymphatic drainage. This blockage may cause lymphedema (peau d'orange skin), which can clinically appear like a malignancy. The dying worms cause an inflammatory reaction, forming a mass with eosinophilic and granulomatous inflammation, which can be chronic. The chronic inflammation may also result in a bacterial infection, in addition to the other changes in the breast.

Myiasis

This is caused by infection from the larvae of flies from the order diptera. When infecting humans, the larvae of these flies usually occupies the skin and subcutis, but can potentially occupy any organ, including the breasts. The human botfly (*Dermatobia hominis*) is the most common of these types of flies, and is found in Central America, South America, and the United States. The tumbu fly (*Cordylobia anthropophaga*) is common in Nigeria. The larvae must feed on the host to complete its development. The infection happens when adult flies use the body openings, such as open wounds or soiled clothes, to lay eggs. Once the botfly larvae get in the skin, it grows to maturity and a nodule/furuncle forms within a few weeks. If infected, you may experience fever, bleeding, and abscess formation. This too can present similar to breast cancer. Treatment involves removing the larvae. Prevention includes good personal hygiene, washing clothes regularly, and possibly ironing clothes after drying them.

Cysticercosis

This is a parasitic worm infection in the breast caused by cysticercosis cellulose. Humans can get this infection from contaminated water or uncooked vegetables. The eggs move to a person's stomach and then move on to other locations when they become larvae, such as the muscles, brain fat tissues, and (rarely) the breast. You can avoid this by treating water and making sure that all food is cooked thoroughly, when living in or visiting an area where this parasite is endemic.

Schistosomiasis

This infection is caused by a parasitic worm that rarely affects the breast. However, if you live in or have travelled to an area where these worms live and you find a lump in your breast, this should be considered as a possible cause. The worms may also be seen on evaluation of the urine or feces, depending on which subtype it is. Adult stages of *S. mansoni, S. japonicum, S. mekongi,* and *S. intercalatum* live in the gut blood supply (mesenteric venous plexus) of infected hosts and the eggs are shed in feces. *S. haematobium* adult worms reside in in the bladder blood supply (venous plexus of the lower urinary tract) and its eggs are shed in urine. When a person has this infection, microcalcifications can be seen in a breast mammogram. This may also be diagnosed with fine needle aspiration.

Yeast Infections

Yeast is a fungus that can affect the breasts and/or the nipples. This occurs more commonly in ladies that are breastfeeding and exposed to thrush (yeast from the infant's mouth) but it can also happen in mothers who are not breastfeeding. Yeast can cause these areas to be painful to touch; even a shower or bath may be painful. The breasts may also feel itchy. When a physician examines the breasts, the skin is sometimes "weeping." It may appear red and irritated. If the area is sampled, you may be able to find yeast. Your healthcare provider would likely encourage you to keep the area dry and treat it with an antifungal medication. Sometimes, there may be another bacterial infection present at the same time, which would require an antibiotic.

Lupus Mastitis

Lupus is a disease where the body's tissues and cells are damaged by its own overactive immune system. Lupus mastitis happens in some patients that have an established diagnosis of lupus. In some cases, it is the mastitis that enables the patient to be diagnosed with this disease. Lupus mastitis can also be the result of lupus panniculitis, which is when nodules (lumps of tissue) occur in the fat of various body parts, including the breasts. In this instance, there may be a single nodule or multiple nodules that can be painful.

The nodules may also turn into ulcers. This is not easy to diagnose, as the signs and imaging can mimic cancer. A substantial biopsy is needed in order to tell this apart from cancer. Once the diagnosis is made, the appropriate treatment can be given to prevent further damage.

Tips to Avoid Mastitis

- Ensure good hand hygiene—wash your hands before touching your breasts.
- Keep the breasts as dry as possible.
- Keep the nipples dry.
- If you are breastfeeding, check to make sure the baby is latching on properly to avoid cracks in the breast.
- Ensure that any member of the family who has a yeast infection is treated.
- Wear cotton bras.
- Ensure the clothing that comes in contact with the breasts has been washed in hot soapy water. Consider drying this clothing using heat or ironing after drying them.
- If you have been in or travelling to a worm or parasite infected area, discuss with your provider.
- Eat a balanced and healthy diet.

Tips to Cope with Mastitis

- Use a warm compress on the affected breast to help with the pain.
- You can use an anti-inflammatory medication, such as Tylenol or Panadol to help.
- Increase fluids and get rest so that your breast has time to repair and heal.
- Massage the breast.
- Allow the breast to be exposed to the sun for 15 minutes a day.
- Seek help to get treatment.

Summary Points

- Your chest may hurt. The pain may or may not be related to your period.
- One of your breasts may be bigger than the other (asymmetry).
- You may have lumps and bumps in your breasts.
- Infections in the breast should be evaluated by a professional and treated immediately.

CHAPTER 11
BREAST PAIN (MASTODYNIA)

Psalm 147:3 (KJV)

*He healeth the broken in heart, and
bindeth up their wounds.*

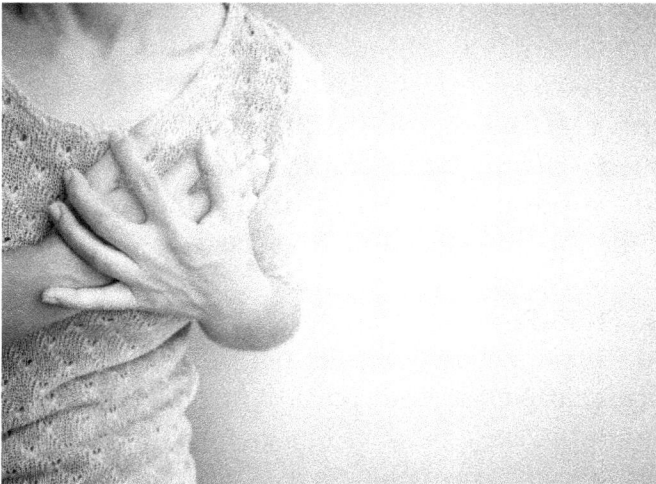

Figure 24 Breast and Chest Wall Pain

Pain in Breast (Matodynia/Mastalgia)

The majority of women will experience breast pain at some point in their lives. Breast pain can make you to feel anxious and it can be complicated. The good news is that most breast pain is not related to cancer. Breast pain may be in one breast (unilateral) or it may be in both (bilateral). It may be related to your period (cyclic) or not related to your period (non-cyclic).

Cyclic Breast Pain (Period Related), Premenstrual Syndrome (PMS), or Premenstrual Dysphoric Disorder (PMDD)

Each month, before their period starts, some ladies have symptoms such as breast tenderness or pain. These symptoms tend to start in the luteal phase of the menstrual cycle and resolve with menstruation. In other words, the symptoms come four to five days before the period starts and stop by the fourth day of the period. The symptoms then remain absent until the next luteal phase. This is called premenstrual syndrome (PMS) or premenstrual dysphoric disorder (PMDD).

The physical (somatic) symptoms of PMS or PMDD may include weight gain, breast tenderness, stomach bloating, joint pain, headaches, nausea, or vomiting. If your breast pain is related to your cycle, you may find that it happens around day 21, when the level of progesterone is at its highest.

PMS and PMDD symptoms can also be emotional (affective), such as confusion, irritability, mood swings, outbursts, anxiety, depression, or withdrawal. This may affect your quality of life and ability to function in your daily activities.

Non-Cyclic (Non-Period) Related Pain

If your pain is not related to your period, it could be caused by conditions that affect the body parts close to the breast, such as inflammation of the chest muscles (costochondritis) or the cartilage and joints (Tietze syndrome).

Costochondritis

Costochondritis is an inflammatory process. You may feel the pain move to your shoulder or arm. The symptoms are similar to symptoms of a heart attack, so it is important to review this with your health care provider.

Tietze Syndrome

Tietze syndrome is a swelling of the joints and cartilage that causes pain where the upper ribs attach to the sternum. The second and third ribs are most commonly affected. Usually, it will feel painful when you press the area or take a deep breath. The pain may come on slowly or suddenly. The pain may also radiate to your shoulders or arms. Your healthcare provider may recommend imaging, but treatment usually involves anti-inflammatory agents and rest. With time, it will usually improve and go away.

Occasionally, pain that is near the breast may be caused by other issues, such as a pulled muscle, gallstones (deposits of solid material in the gallbladder), or angina (chest pain caused by reduced blood flow and oxygen to the heart). These issues may cause inflammation inside of the body that then lead to chest pain.

You may also have breast pain as the side effect of a medication you are taking, such as birth control pills, hormone replacement therapy, infertility treatments, antidepressants, blood pressure medications, steroids, and some heart medications. You should also check to make sure your bra is fitting properly.

If you are experiencing breast pain, your health care provider may ask you to keep a diary for two months to document it. They will have you document the severity and type of pain, such as whether it is shooting, stabbing, sharp, heavy, tender, crampy, throbbing, etc. You may be asked to describe the pattern of the pain, such as whether it comes and goes or is constant. It is also important to document whether it affects your sleep, work, and sex life. You should also document whether you have pain in one or both breasts, and whether medications help alleviate the pain. All of this information will help your health care provider understand the pain better, especially because you may not remember everything when you see the heath care provider. Studies (ARJ 2018) have shown that most women who report chest pain have a negative study (nothing bad was found) when imaged with mammogram. Most cases will also resolve spontaneously. So, if you have chest pain, do not be alarmed if your health care provider does not rush to order an imaging study.

When trying to find a treatment regimen, you'll likely need to try different interventions. Diet changes, such as decreasing caffeine intake, reducing salt intake, and taking some vitamins such as Vitamin E, B6, B1, and evening primrose oil may be helpful in reducing the pain. Herbal supplements such as chasteberry may also be beneficial. Exercise, decreasing stress, and maintaining a healthy weight may also decrease pain.

You can also try wearing a supportive sports bra, keeping your stress level down, and taking over-the-counter pain medications (as directed). In severe cases, Tamoxifen (an estrogen modulator) may be used as well. Discuss this issue with your health care provider, who can examine you and help get to the root of the problem.

Summary Points

- Breast pain is experienced by many women.
- Breast pain should be brought to the attention of your health care provider.
- Breast pain may be on one side or both sides.
- Breast pain may be cyclic (related to your menstrual cycle) or non-cyclic.
- Lifestyle modifications may play a role in helping to address breast pain if is related to the breast tissue.
- Breast pain may be caused by a problem with areas that are close to the breasts, such as the heart or the chest wall.

CHAPTER 12

NIPPLE DISCHARGE

❧

Jeremiah 17:14 (NIV)

Heal me, Lord, and I will be healed;
save me and I will be saved,
for you are the one I praise.

Nipple Discharge

Nipple discharge is a common complaint. It refers to any discharge that comes out of the nipples. The discharge can be spontaneous and it may come from one or both sides. Sometimes it is the result of pregnancy or a post-pregnancy state. Sometimes it happens during stimulation of the breast. Nipple discharge is of concern when it is persistent and happens when you are not stimulating the breast.

Nipple discharge can have any color. Below is a summary of different types, colors, and contents of nipple discharge.

Table 7

Types of Nipple Discharge	Features
Milky	Discharge is white; fat globules may be seen if you look at it under the microscope.
Watery	Discharge without color.
Multicolored gummous	Sticky discharge.
Purulent	Yellow or green, may be malodorous. Contains dead white blood cells, bacteria, and serum, which can be seen under the microscope.
Bloody	Red blood cells (RBCs) can be seen under the microscope.
Serous	Thin, faintly yellow discharge.
Serosanguinous	Thin, clear discharge with a pink tint. RBCs can be seen under the microscope.

Discharge that is related to a non-cancerous condition is usually milky. This type is not purulent or bloody. This can be caused by a number of things, such as medication, stimulation of the breast, pregnancy or being postpartum, having a recent miscarriage, or having a problem with your hormone producing glands such as the thyroid or pituitary gland.

Purulent discharge may be from an infection, as discussed in the section on mastitis. (See chapter on mastitis.) Bloody discharge may be a result of fibrocystic changes, problems with the nipple(s) or glands of the breast, and problems in the breast tissue, such as cancer. (See chapter on breast cancer.)

Some medications may cause discharge from the breast. These medications include the following:

- Birth control pills.
- Medications for nausea, such as metoclopramide.
- Medications for blood pressure, such as methyldopa, verapamil, and reserpine.
- Medications used to stabilize mood, such as butyrophenones and phenothiazines.

- Medication for pain, such as cannabinoids and opiates (marijuana, morphine, heroin).

Table 8 Causes of Nipple Discharge and Associated Color

Causes of Nipple Discharge	Color of the Discharge
Hypothyroidism	White
Galactorrhea	White or green
Intraductal papilloma	Bloody
Periductal mastitis	White, cloudy, or yellow (pus like)
Ductal ectasia	Brown or orange/yellow

Galactorrhea
Galactorrhea is defined as milk discharge from the breasts when you are not breastfeeding or postpartum. This usually involves multiple duct discharge from both breasts. The cause of galactorrhea is usually a prolactin abnormality. Galactorrhea associated with high prolactin can be caused by failure of the normal hypothalamic inhibition of prolactin release, enhanced prolactin-releasing factor, or autonomous or ectopic prolactin-releasing factor.

Lesions (such as tumors) found in the hypothalamus or pituitary stalk, or drugs that influence the central nervous system, can decrease the inhibitory dopaminergic control of prolactin. A physiologic enhancement of prolactin release is caused by thyrotropin releasing hormone. Three types of pituitary tumors may be associated with galactorrhea: pure prolactin-secreting tumors (microadenoma or macroadenoma), mixed tumors that secrete both growth hormone and prolactin, and chromophobe adenomas. Prolactin can also (rarely) be secreted by other malignancies, such as lung cancer (bronchogenic carcinoma), hydatidiform moles, choriocarcinomas, and kidney cancer (hypernephromas). Some ladies with galactorrhea will have an increase in prolactin levels, but the majority of patients will have normal prolactin levels.

Table 9 Causes of Galactorrhea

Hyperprolactinemic galactorrhea	Physiologic	Tumors	Lesions involving chest wall	Systemic Disease
Hypothalamic or infundibular lesions • Craniopharyngioma • Germinoma • Meningioma • Rathke's cleft cysts	Nipple manipulation	Pituitary lesions	Breast surgery	Hypothyroidism
Infiltrative disorders • Sarcoidosis • Histiocytosis	Breast manipulation	Prolactinoma	Trauma	Herpes zoster
Medication-induced hyperprolactinemia	Pregnancy	Growth hormone secreting tumors, acromegaly	Burns	Renal insufficiency
Other Choriocarcinoma	Breastfeeding	Null cell tumors	Lung cancer	Idiopathic hyperprolactinemia
		Breast Cancer	Kidney tumor	Spinal cord injury

Primary Hypothyroidism

The thyroid gland in the front of the neck makes hormones that control metabolism (the way your body burns energy). Primary hypothyroidism results in increases of thyroid releasing hormone, which can cause prolactin release and galactorrhea. This can be cured with thyroid hormone replacement therapy.

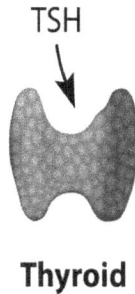

TSH

Thyroid

Figure 25 Thyroid Stimulating Effect on Thyroid Gland

Breast Surgery/Breast Trauma

Breast surgery or trauma can result in an enhanced secretion of oxytocin. It is also thought that the trauma or surgery may interfere with nerve innovation in this area, thereby affecting the hypothalamic (master gland) control over milk secretions.

Intraductal Papilloma and Papillomatosis

Intraductal papilloma usually presents as a spontaneous (without stimulation) and intermittent bloody discharge from one nipple in a woman that is perimenopausal. The discharge may have varying consistency, from watery to bloody.

An intraductal papilloma is a wart-like, benign tumor of the mammary ducts. It can appear anywhere in the breast ducts but is often found at the ends of the ducts underneath the nipple. These can appear in one area or multiple. If you have five or more papilloma, this is called papillomatosis. It is referred to as juvenile papillomatosis when it is found in women under 30 years old. Having multiple papillomas can increase the risk of breast cancer. A single papilloma without atypical cells does not increase risk. Treatment involves excising the area of concern.

Periductal Mastitis/Ductal ectasia
Periductal mastitis (also known as ductal ectasia) happens when there is a blockage in the subareolar ducts. As a result, you may notice discharge from the nipple, which may be sticky and can vary in color. The nipple may also be itchy and painful. This breast discharge will usually resolve on its own. If it does not, your health care provider may refer you to a surgeon to remove the affected area. This does not increase your risk of cancer.

Advice If You Have Nipple Discharge
If you have nipple discharge that persists, you should see your health care provider. They will review your family and medical history, as discussed in chapter two. They will also perform a physical exam. The provider may order laboratory tests, such as those that look at your thyroid and prolactin levels. They may ask you to get additional testing and an ultrasound to help figure out why you are having the discharge.

Workup of Breast Discharge
This discharge workup may include testing, such as a pregnancy test, thyroid test, and checking the prolactin hormone (which plays a role in milk secretion). Your provider may also order tests to check your liver and kidney. A mammogram and/or breast ultrasound may be requested. (See chapter on breast imaging.) Sometimes they may also do a ductoscopy, which is a procedure that gathers information and looks closely at the ducts in the breast.

Treatment of Breast Discharge

The treatment of breast discharge will be determined by its cause. If the cause is something related to a lesion in the breast, the lesion may need to be removed. If the discharge if due to an infection, it can be treated with antibiotics. Discharge caused by a high hormone level (prolactin) will likely be treated with medication. If a medication you are already taking is causing the discharge, you may need to stop or change the medication. If the discharge is due to a brain tumor, this may be monitored or need to be removed. However, in some cases the cause is not determined (idiopathic). These cases may be more of a challenge to treat.

Summary Points

- Nipple discharge is a common symptom that should be brought to the attention of your health care provider.
- Different causes may produce different colors of discharge.
- Hormonal testing may be needed to find out the cause.
- If the cause is determined, a treatment course will be designed to address the underlying reason.

CHAPTER 13

SKIN DISORDERS
OF THE BREASTS

❧

Jeremiah 30:17 (KJV)

*For I will restore health unto thee, and I will heal thee of
thy wounds, saith the Lord; because they called thee an
Outcast, saying, This is Zion, whom no man seeketh after.*

Intertrigo (Rash Under the Breast)
Intertrigo (sometimes called candidal intertrigo) is a common
condition that causes a rash between the folds of skin under one
or both breasts. The main causes of intertrigo include friction between the skin folds, heat, and moisture. This results in a rash that
may be reddish or brown. The skin may be cracked, and the area
may be raw and weeping. The person may or may not have pain.

Intertrigo can occur anywhere on the body where skin rubs
against skin, such as between the thighs or on the underside of the
belly or armpit. A warm, moist environment encourages infection

by either yeast, fungus, or bacteria. Sometimes swelling, sores and blisters can also occur.

If you think you have intertrigo, speak to your health care provider. They will exam the area and make recommendations based on what they suspect is the underlying cause. The goals of treatment would be as follows:

- Treat any infection and prevent it from spreading
- Reduce the rubbing of skin on skin
- Keep the area dry and free of moisture
- Reduce inflammation

You can reduce your risk of getting intertrigo and stop any irritation from getting worse by trying the following steps:

1. Losing weight, which will limit the areas where skin can rub against skin.
2. Wash under your breasts in the morning and night with a gentle soap or soap substitute (for example, with an ointment that acts as a skin protectant against moisture).
3. Dry the skin under your breasts after washing. Gently pat dry with a clean, soft towel or use a fan or hairdryer on a cool setting.
4. Wear a bra that fits well and gives proper support. (See chapter on fitting a bra.)
5. Treatments such as barrier creams, steroid creams, antifungal creams, and antibiotic creams or tablets may also help. You can ask your doctor or pharmacist about these.

Breast Acne
Acne is an inflammatory skin disease that affects the skin follicles. This can occur on the chest or breasts. If you have acne on your breasts, you can use the same acne products that you use on your

face on the breast area. Keep the chest clean. If antibiotics are required, they can be applied topically, or they may be used systemically (taken orally). A dermatologist (a doctor specializing in skin conditions) may be helpful in managing this issue.

Allergic or Contact Dermatitis of the Breasts
If you are exposed to a chemical or substance that irritates the breasts, it may cause a reaction in the skin. If a certain product causes skin irritation, you may have irritant contact dermatitis. It is considered an allergy when you have an allergic reaction to a product that is used on the skin.

Eczema of the Breasts
Eczema happens when the outside layer of your skin gets inflamed when exposed to external bacteria, allergens, and irritants. Atopic dermatitis is the most common form of eczema. Breast eczema may affect the nipples, areolae, or surrounding skin. Eczema of the nipples tends to be the moist type (with oozing and crusting) in which painful fissuring is frequently seen, especially in nursing mothers. It will often occur in pregnancy, even without breastfeeding. We do not know the exact reason breast eczema happens. We do understand that if you or your family has a history of eczema, hay fever, or asthma, your risk of eczema increases.

Eczema on the breasts is one of the most common causes of breast itchiness. Breakouts can also occur under or in-between your breasts, and on the rest of your chest. While symptoms can vary, you may experience:

- Dry, cracked, itching skin
- Red or brownish-gray areas of skin under, in-between, or on your breasts
- Small bumps that may discharge fluid and crust over after repeated scratching
- Swelling due to scratching

To avoid breakouts:

- Wash the breasts well
- Avoid hot showers
- Avoid soaps, shampoos, perfumes, or body products on the breasts—especially the nipple area
- Do not use bras with pads because the padding can hold on to the chemicals that are irritating the breasts
- Wash bras with a simple hypoallergenic soap

Treatment
One method of treatment is to use prescription steroid ointments. You would apply the ointment to the affected area, once or twice daily, for seven days. If you are breastfeeding, apply the ointment sparingly after a feed. After seven days, switch to a 1% hydrocortisone ointment applied once daily.

Acanthosis Nigricans
This is skin condition that may be the result of other systemic illnesses, such as diabetes, hormonal imbalances, thyroid disease, cancer, and obesity. It may also be caused by certain medications, such as birth control pills. In acanthosis nigricans, the areas where the body folds or creases (such as underneath the breasts) may appear discolored and thickened. The area may also be dry and itchy. Treatment involves treating the underlying cause.

Tinea Versicolor (Pityriasis Versicolor or "Shifting Clouds")
This is a fungal infection that can affect the breasts. The affected areas have defined margins and the skin often appears lighter than the surrounding normal skin. These lesions are usually located on the trunk, including at the top of the breasts and the space in-between the breasts. This infection happens in areas of the body that are warm and moist, especially in the summer months. Treatment involves the use of azole antifungal medications or sulfides. As this

may have a high risk of recurrence and can appear similar to other skin disorders, it is best to see a dermatologist (skin specialist) for an expert opinion and treatment regimen.

Scabies of the Breasts

Scabies are mites that live on the surface of the skin. They like warm places, including the breasts. The most common symptoms of scabies include extreme itchiness (which is worse at night) and rash. The rash may look like it has blisters. Scabies is treated by using permethrin or lindane to kill the mites.

Seborrheic Dermatitis

This is an inflammatory skin condition that can affect different parts of the body, including the breasts. Symptoms of seborrheic dermatitis include a rash, itchy skin, greasy skin patches, or dandruff. This may be caused by a response of the immune system (autoimmune response). Sometimes a sample of the area or a biopsy is done to confirm the diagnosis.

One way to improve the outcome of seborrheic dermatitis is to take good care of your skin. You can also use your diet to help by avoiding foods that may cause inflammation. (See breast health and foods chapter.) The use of any of the following may act as an anti-inflammatory to help prevent flare ups:

- Probiotics
- Fish oil
- Aloe vera
- Tea tree oil

This condition is chronic and may come and go. Treatment can help control the flare ups. Seek out care and advice from a health care provider early.

Psoriasis of the Breasts

Psoriasis is an autoimmune condition that may result in patches that appear on the skin, including on the breasts. There are a variety of symptoms, including red, inflamed skin or scaly patches. These areas may itch, sting, or burn. It is important to have this condition assessed by a medical professional, as some cases are found in people with breast cancer. This condition may make it more challenging to breastfeed.

A small percentage of people with psoriasis have inverse psoriasis (also known as intertriginous psoriasis). This causes red and inflamed lesions in the skin folds, including under the breasts. People who are overweight or have deep skin folds have a higher chance of developing this type of psoriasis.

Hidradenitis Suppurativa

Hidradenitis suppurativa is a chronic skin disease which is characterized by pea-sized lumps and bumps that come and go. These lumps develop on the skin near the hair follicles and can be painful. Being a smoker or being overweight can increase your chance of having this issue.

It is thought that anaerobic actinomyces may play a role in this disease process. Your health care provider may use diet, antibiotics, and other medications to try to prevent long-term damage to the tissue. Quitting smoking, losing any extra weight, wearing loose fitting clothing, and maintaining a healthy diet may help decrease the severity of outbreaks.

Summary Points

- Skin disorders of the breasts may happen.
- Keep the breasts clean and dry.
- Wear clothes that do not irritate the breasts.
- Eat a healthy diet.
- Quit any social activities that may negatively affect the breasts, such as smoking or alcohol use.
- Decrease your stress.
- Seek dermatologic (skin) or breast specialist care if a skin issue persists.

CHAPTER 14

OTHER DISEASES THAT
AFFECT THE BREAST

❧

Matthew 9:12 (KJV)

*But when Jesus heard that, he said unto them, they that be
whole need not a physician, but they that are sick.*

There are a variety of systemic disorders like diabetes, sarcoidosis, vascular disease, shingles, and amyloidosis that can affect the breasts along with the rest of the body. In some cases, the effects of the illness may initially be noticed in the breasts.

Endocrine Disorders

Diabetes and the Breasts
Diabetes can affect the breasts. For example, diabetic fibrous mastopathy can happen if you have long standing Type I or Type II diabetes, especially if you've had other complications. You may have a single lump or multiple lumps in the breasts that feel firm but

painless. The lumps are caused by an inflammatory increase in the breast tissue. As the findings of mastopathy on imaging can appear similar to malignancy, a biopsy may be needed to show that it is noncancerous. Diabetes can also cause acanthosis nigricans (thickened skin under the breasts).

Sarcoidosis of the Breast
Sarcoidosis is an inflammatory disease that affects many systems in the body, including the breasts. It may involve the breast parenchyma and create lesions that can be confused with benign or malignant tumors. The mean age that people present with sarcoidosis is in their forties. Some patients have a breast mass as primary presentation of sarcoidosis without any clinical evidence of systemic sarcoidosis (masses appearing in other parts of the body). The breast lesions may vary. It commonly only affects one breast but can also affect both.

Mammography and ultrasound can be used to aid in diagnosis, but sampling the tissue through fine needle aspiration, core biopsy, or excisional biopsy may give a more definitive diagnosis when a sarcoid granuloma is found.

Pseudoangiomatous Stromal Hyperplasia (PASH)
PASH is a type of noncancerous breast lesion. When a person has this disorder, the affected breast may or may not rapidly enlarge. It typically affects women in the reproductive age group, but it can also affect children, adolescents, and postmenopausal women. Often this is found when you are not looking for it (incidentally) when a sample of the breast (biopsy) is done. If diagnosed with PASH, your health care provider would review treatment options with you, which may include just watching the area (observation), or the use of a laser or other means to remove the lesion (surgical excision).

Juvenile (Virginal) Breast Hypertrophy

Juvenile breast hypertrophy occurs in prepubertal females. The exact cause is unknown. It can lead to a rapid enlargement of the breasts which can result in back or neck pain. The blood vessels in the breasts may also increase in size. Treatment may require a removal of an area of the breasts.

Vascular Disease

Some diseases affect your blood vessels, causing a decrease in blood flow. This can be caused by end-stage renal disease or cardiovascular disease. The decrease in blood flow can result in the dying and breaking down of tissue. The findings of this may look like a malignancy in the breasts, so a biopsy may be needed to make the diagnosis.

Giant Cell Arteritis

This a rare vascular disease that may affect the breasts. It can cause redness and tenderness in the breasts, with or without lumps. In many cases, the diagnosis is only made after the area is excised (removed).

Granulomatosis with Polyangiitis (GPA), Formerly Known as Wegner's Disease

GPA is an inflammation of the small and medium blood vessels (vasculitis) in the body. In rare cases, this disease can affect the breasts, typically in ladies between 30-70 years old. It may show up as a lesion in one or both breasts. Due to inflammation in the breast tissue, it may present with symptoms similar to breast cancer, granulomatous mastitis, a breast abscess, or an ulceration. Mammogram and ultrasound can be used to help evaluate the breasts. Once adequate tissue is sampled, a breast biopsy is helpful in making the diagnosis. The treatment may involve the use of immunosuppressants or removing the area.

Polyarteritis Nodosa

This is a vascular disease that rarely affects the breasts, but it can mimic breast cancer or infections of the breast. The good thing is that it can be diagnosed on biopsy. If present, it can be treated by suppressing the immune system. Sometimes the affected area may need to be removed (debrided) to take out the unhealthy tissue.

Shingles of the Breast

Shingles is a viral infection caused by the varicella zoster virus, which is a type of herpes virus. This group includes the viruses that cause cold sores, genital herpes, and chickenpox. The virus affects the nerves. Once infected with the virus, it does not go away. It remains in the nerve tissue near your spinal cord and brain. If the virus reactivates, it can cause shingles.

Shingles usually affects a small section of one side of your body. The most common signs and symptoms are:

- Pain, burning, numbness, or tingling
- Tiredness
- Headache
- Fever
- Sensitivity to touch or sensitivity to light
- A red rash
- Fluid-filled blisters that break open and crust over
- Itching

Anyone who has ever had chickenpox can develop shingles. Most adults in the Bahamas have had chickenpox when they were children, before the advent of the routine childhood vaccination that now protects against chickenpox.

Vaccines are available that may help prevent shingles—the chickenpox (varicella) vaccine and the shingles (varicella zoster) vaccine. The varicella vaccine has become a routine childhood immunization to prevent chickenpox. The vaccine is also recommended for adults who've never had chickenpox. Though the vaccine doesn't guarantee that you won't get chickenpox or shingles, it can reduce your chances of complications from the illness, such as postherpetic neuralgia. It can also reduce the severity of the disease. Please discuss with your health care provider whether this vaccine would benefit you.

Shingles is most common in people over 50, people with chronic diseases that weaken the immune system, people receiving cancer treatment, or those on medications that suppress the immune system. Contact your health provider if you suspect that you have shingles. Early treatment may help shorten a shingles infection and lessen the chance of complications.

Diffuse Dermal Angiomatosis

This is a condition where the blood vessels cause lesions that are painful and purple. The lesions tend to be non-healing and may affect both breasts. They are more commonly found on the underside of the breasts. This is usually diagnosed with a sample of the area, called a punch biopsy. Once the diagnosis is made, medication may be recommended that can be helpful.

Amyloidosis of the Breast

This is a rare disease that may be found in persons who have systemic amyloidosis, or it may just be found in the breast. It may present as skin thickening or a lesion in the breast. The amyloid in the breast may cause a foreign body type of reaction. Treatment involves removing the area of concern.

Summary Points

- Diseases that affect other body systems may either present in the breasts or manifest in the breasts.
- Some of the systemic manifestations of diseases can be difficult to distinguish from malignancy (cancer).
- Imaging may be helpful in diagnosing these issues.
- Review by a specialist and tissue sampling are important in helping to make a diagnosis.
- Once the diagnosis is made, the best treatment pathway can be decided upon.

SECTION III
CANCER, IMAGING, BREAST PROCEDURES, AND SURGERIES

❧

CHAPTER 15

RISK FACTORS FOR BREAST CANCER

❧

Isaiah 60:16 (KJV)

*Thou shalt also suck the milk of the Gentiles,
and shalt suck the breast of kings: and thou
shalt know that I the Lord am thy Saviour and
thy Redeemer, the mighty One of Jacob.*

Breast cancer is a complicated disease process. It is a concern for both males and females but is more common in women than in men. It is the most common cancer in women worldwide. The risk of breast cancer increases with age. If it's found early, it may be easier to treat, with improved outcomes and a better survival rate.

Risk Factors for Breast Cancer
A risk factor is anything about you that puts you at an increased chance for having a disease. Risk factors are thought to identify one out of four women who will develop breast cancer. Some of these

factors are modifiable, meaning you can change them. Others are due to genetics, and therefore cannot be changed.

Table 10 Modifiable and Non-Modifiable Risk Factors for Breast Cancer

Modifiable Risk Factors	Non-Modifiable Risk Factors
• Obesity	• Age
• Alcohol consumption	• Gender
• Diet	• Density of breasts
• Age at first pregnancy	• Early age at first menstruation
• Hormone replacement therapy	• Personal history of breast disease with or without atypia
• Oral birth control	• Personal history of rheumatologic disorders
• Exposure to radiation	• Family history of breast cancer or breast disease
	• Juvenile papillomatosis
	• Benign breast disease

Age: Breast cancer risk increases with age. We often say there is a one in eight chance that a woman will develop breast cancer in her lifetime. However, it is important to understand that this risk is based on a lady who is age 90. A woman in her 30's has a risk of 1 in 227. At age 60, the risk increases to 1 in 28.

Gender: Females are more likely than males to get breast cancer. Women in the western world have a higher risk than women in other parts of the world. Transgender females have an increased risk of breast cancer which is thought to be related to the use of hormones.

Obesity: As your weight increases, it causes the amount of estrogen in your body to rise, which increases your breast cancer risk. The increase in fat means that there is a higher peripheral conversion of androstenedione to estrogen and lower levels of sex-hormone binding globulin.

Breast Density: Density refers to how the breasts look on mammogram. The connective tissue and ducts give the breasts a solid appearance, whereas fatty tissue looks clear and transparent. Having dense breasts means an increased risk for breast cancer. Dense breasts also make it more difficult to take imaging.

Personal history of any type of cancer: If you have had any other type of cancer, this may increase your risk of developing breast cancer. This increased risk may be because of how your body is made up or it may be because of the treatment that you underwent. If you have had breast cancer in one breast, this may increase the chance of developing cancer in the other breast.

Family history of breast disease: If you have a first degree relative (e.g., mother, sister, daughter) who has had breast disease this may increase your risk.

Family history of breast cancer: If you have a first degree relative (e.g., a sister or mother) that has had breast cancer, this may increase your risk.

Personal history of breast disease with or without atypia: These increase your risk of breast cancer and more aggressive breast cancer types:

- Radial adenosis
- Ductal lobular hyperplasia
- Peripheral intraductal papillomas
- Radial scars
- Fibromatosis
- Flat epithelial atypia
- Benign phyllodes tumor
- Juvenile papillomatosis

Early age at first menstruation: This increases the amount of time that you have been exposed to estrogen, which can increase your risk of breast cancer.

Hormone replacement therapy or oral birth control pills: These medications increase the amount of estrogen that your body is exposed to. The exact mechanism is not fully understood, but it is thought that women who are using combination estrogen and progesterone pills have a higher risk than women who are using hormonal replacement regimens with estrogen only.

Exposure to radiation: If you have been exposed to radiation early in life, such as to treat cancer, lymphoma, an enlarged thymus, or acne, you may have an increased risk of breast cancer—particularly angiosarcoma.

Risk reduction is when you do things to decrease the chance that you will develop breast cancer. Certain risk reduction activities have been shown to significantly decrease your risk, sometimes by as much as 18–30% or more. Risk reduction activities involve the following:

- Exercising regularly.
- Maintaining a healthy weight.
- Eating lots of fruits and vegetables and whole grain foods.
- Limiting foods with preservatives.
- Limiting meat intake and opting for meat that that has not been exposed to chemicals.
- Choosing polyunsaturated and monounsaturated fats over saturated and trans fats.
- Limiting alcohol intake.
- Limiting menopausal hormone therapy.
- Having children, if that is an option for you.
- Breastfeeding, if that is an option for you.

There are certain characteristics about you that you may not be able to change—called non-modifiable risk factors—that increase your chance of having an abnormality, such as age.

Tumor Suppressor Genes
Genes are found in each cell of your body. They provide a blueprint or coding for the proteins that your body builds. BRCA genes are normal genes that function to prevent tumor formation (tumor suppressors). They repair DNA damage in your cells, thereby preventing cancer. Each of your cells contains two copies of each BRCA gene (BRCA1 and BRCA2)—one copy from each parent. Mutations affect the gene's ability to carry out its normal function. A mutation may be inherited (passed down from one parent) or acquired as a result of DNA damage related to the environment, lifestyle factors (like smoking), or even normal metabolic processes in cells. Certain inherited mutations in BRCA genes can lead to an increased risk of breast cancer.

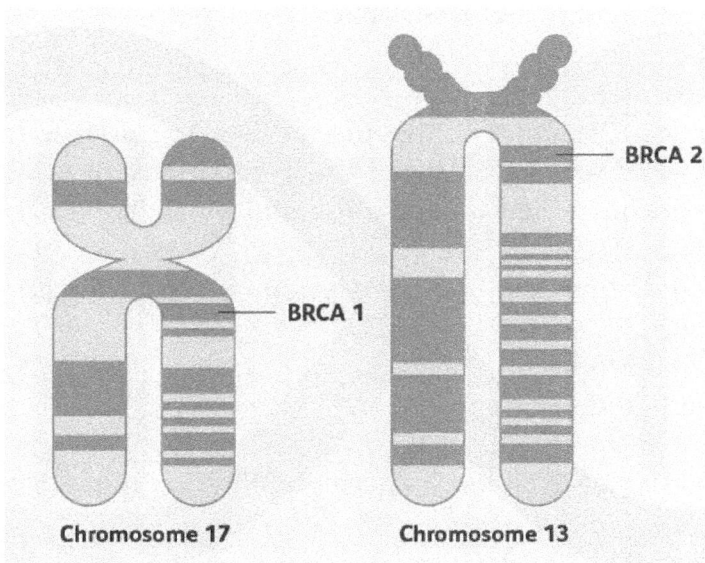

Figure Location of BRCA Genes on Chromosomes 17 and 13

BRCA 1

- More common that BRCA 2
- Located on Chromosome 17q21.3
- Tends to develop more aggressive tumors that have a worse predicted outcome (prognosis)
- Cancers present at a younger age
- Lifetime breast cancer risk of 60-70%
- Lifetime ovarian cancer risk of 40-50%

BRCA 2

- Chromosome 13q12-13
- Cancers are similar to patients that do not have BRCA genes
- Lifetime breast cancer risk is 40-50%
- Lifetime ovarian cancer risk is 10-12%

New genetic mutations are being discovered regularly. Some of the more common ones are listed below.

Risk Assessment

There are different models that may be used to calculate your lifetime risk of breast cancer, BRCA1 or 2 mutations, or other breast cancer syndromes. See appendix for additional details.

Models predicting likelihood of developing breast cancer:

- Claus Model
- Gail Model

Models predicting likelihood of having a BRCA1 or BRCA2 mutation:

- Myriad risk tables
- Couch

- Shattuck-Eidens
- CaGene mutations

Model predicting likelihood of breast cancer syndrome:

- Pedigree analysis: This is a study on how we inherit genes

Genetic Testing
Genetic testing is when you look for possible causes of cancer in your genetic makeup. Usually genetic testing is recommended if you have characteristics that put you at an increased risk of developing a cancer that may be genetic. Some of the factors that may cause concern for genetic cancers are below.

Concern about genetic causes of cancer

- Concerns regarding hereditary ovarian cancer
- Breast cancer before age 50
- Ovarian cancer at any age
- Male breast cancer at any age
- Having two primary family members who have had breast cancer at any age
- Having two or more people in the family who have had breast cancer under age 50
- Women of Ashkenazi Jewish ancestry with breast or ovarian cancer at any age
- A previously identified BRCA mutation in the family

If you have an increased genetic risk of cancer, more frequent monitoring is required, and you may be recommended a medication to lower your risk. Sometimes you are offered surgery to try to decrease your risk. For example, it may be recommended that you have your breasts and ovaries removed after childbearing is completed.

Summary Points

- Know what your risk factors for breast cancer are.
- Decrease your risk factors where possible.
- Genetic cases of breast cancer are usually a result of a gene mutation that has been inherited from your parents and/or a mutation caused by your lifestyle or environment.
- Many genetic causes of cancer exist. The more common ones include BRCA1 and BRCA2.
- Get genetic counselling where indicated.

CHAPTER 16

BREAST CANCER AND PRECANCEROUS LESIONS

❧

2 Corinthians 1:3-4 (KJV)

*Blessed be God, even the Father of our Lord Jesus Christ,
the Father of mercies, and the God of all comfort; Who
comforteth us in all our tribulation, that we may be able
to comfort them which are in any trouble, by the comfort
wherewith we ourselves are comforted of God.*

B reast cancer and precancerous lesions are very concerning for many ladies. Worldwide, breast cancer continues to be one of the most common cancers in women. I, as a clinician, cannot express the devastation and sorrow that often follow the words, "the biopsy did not come out well, you have breast cancer." It is like someone has rear ended you in car crash. Although I am not a breast surgeon or an oncologist, as a gynecologist in the Caribbean, I may be your first point of contact. We will refer you to a surgeon or a center that provides a multidisciplinary approach for treatment.

Definition of Precancerous Breast Lesions
These are lesions in the breast that have the potential to change into cancer cells that are either non-invasive (carcinoma in situ) or invasive. There is discussion in the medical community as to whether these lesions are simply a risk factor for cancer or if they definitely occur prior to the cells changing into cancer.

Definition of Breast Cancer
Breast cancer occurs when the normal cells of the breast start to grow in an abnormal way. Initially the abnormal cells may remain confined to the breast tissue, but if left undiagnosed or untreated, they may move from the breast to other organs in the body. Most breast cancers begin in the cells that line the ducts (ductal cancers). Some begin in the cells that line the lobules (lobular cancers). A small number begin in other breast tissues. The majority of breast cancer cases will be confined to the breasts when they are diagnosed.

Symptoms of Breast Cancer
Cancer and noncancerous diseases of the breasts can present with similar signs and symptoms, which can be confusing. Some of these symptoms include:

- No symptoms
- A breast mass
- Changes in the breast skin
- Changes to the lymph nodes under the arms
- Changes to the way the nipple looks
- Nipple discharge
- Fluid in the breast
- Breast pain
- Redness or swelling in the breast

Types of Breast Cancer

The types of breast cancer are named and broken down into groups based on the cells that they originate in.

Table 11 Tumor Type and Related Histologic Subtype

Tumor Location	Histologic Subtype	Information on Subtype
Ductal Carcinoma, NOS (80% of lesions)	Intraductal (*in situ*). The cancer is in its original place, confined to the duct	Confined but can progress to invasive cancer.
	Invasive with predominant intraductal component	May be more likely to be discovered on imaging. It may have a similar prognosis to invasive ductal carcinoma.
	Invasive, NOS	It has spread beyond the duct to other parts of the breast.
	Comedo-type	The dead cells (necrosis) inside the abnormal area looks like a comedo (blackhead).
	Inflammatory	Rapid development. Cancer cells block the lymphatic glands, causing the skin to become red.
	Medullary with lymphocytic infiltrate	A rare cancer.
	Mucinous (colloid)	Begins in the milk duct. Has a good prognosis. Develops in older postmenopausal women.
	Papillary	Develops in older postmenopausal women and men. Presents with bloody discharge.
	Scirrhous	Slow growing tumors that mostly occurs in elderly women.
	Tubular	These tend to be small tumors that are less aggressive. Less likely to recur. Usually luminal A type cancers with a good prognosis.
	Other	N/A

(*Continued*)

Table 11 Tumor Type and Related Histologic Subtype (*Continued*)

Lobular (10-15% of lesions)	Invasive with predominant *in situ* component	This may not have any symptoms or produce a lump.
	Invasive	May be more difficult to see on mammogram. Tends to occur in women ages 45-55.
Nipple	Paget disease, NOS	Affects the nipple-areolar complex. Causes a thickened rash.
	Paget disease with intraductal carcinoma	Affects the nipple-areolar complex. Also linked to intraductal carcinoma.
	Paget disease with invasive ductal carcinoma	Affects the nipple-areolar complex. An invasive type of cancer.
Other	Undifferentiated carcinoma	This cancer is aggressive as the cells have not specialized into a specific cell type. Tends to be harder to treat.
	Metaplastic	Cancer that has moved to the breast from different organs, such as the colon or ovary.

Adenocarcinoma

This is the most common type of breast cancer. Many different types of cancer fall under this category. Adenocarcinoma covers any cancer that starts in the cells that make up your glands (glandular tissue). Breast adenocarcinomas start in the ducts (the milk ducts) or the lobules (milk-producing glands).

BREAST CANCER
DUCTAL CARCINOMA

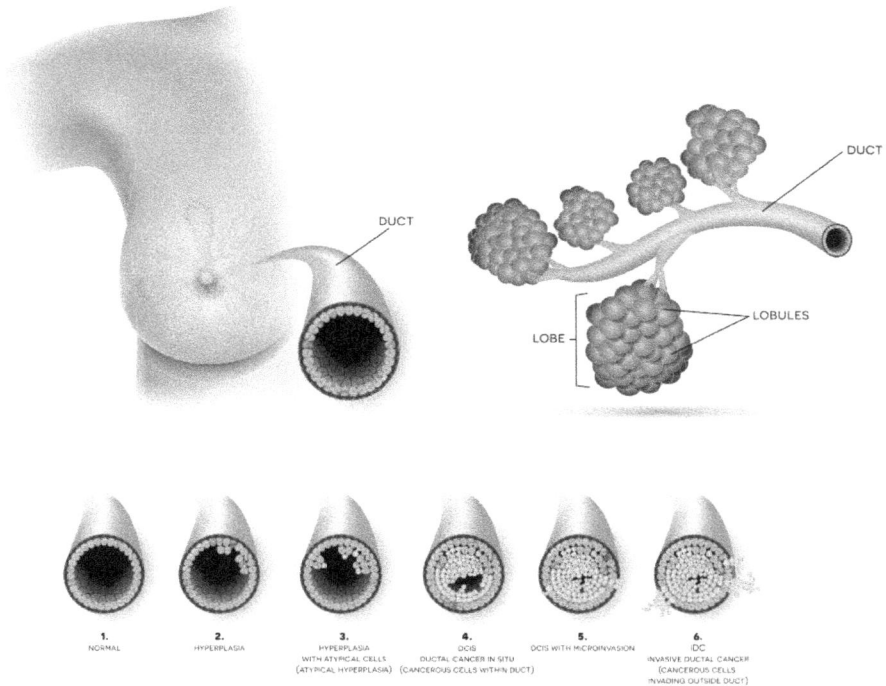

DUCT

DUCT

LOBULES

LOBE

1.	2.	3.	4.	5.	6.
NORMAL	HYPERPLASIA	HYPERPLASIA WITH ATYPICAL CELLS (ATYPICAL HYPERPLASIA)	DCIS DUCTAL CANCER IN SITU (CANCEROUS CELLS WITHIN DUCT)	DCIS WITH MICROINVASION	IDC INVASIVE DUCTAL CANCER (CANCEROUS CELLS INVADING OUTSIDE DUCT)

Figure 26 Ductal Carcinoma Breast Cancer

As seen in image 1, the normal layer contains cells that are in the right place—lining the duct. In image 2, hyperplasia has occurred and there are too many cells lining the duct. Image 3 starts to represent atypia, which is when the cells are becoming abnormal. Image 4 shows the cancer cells are inside the duct (in situ). Image 5 shows how the abnormal cells start to move out of the duct. Image 6 shows invasive ductal cancer, where the cells have moved outside the duct to affect the surrounding tissue.

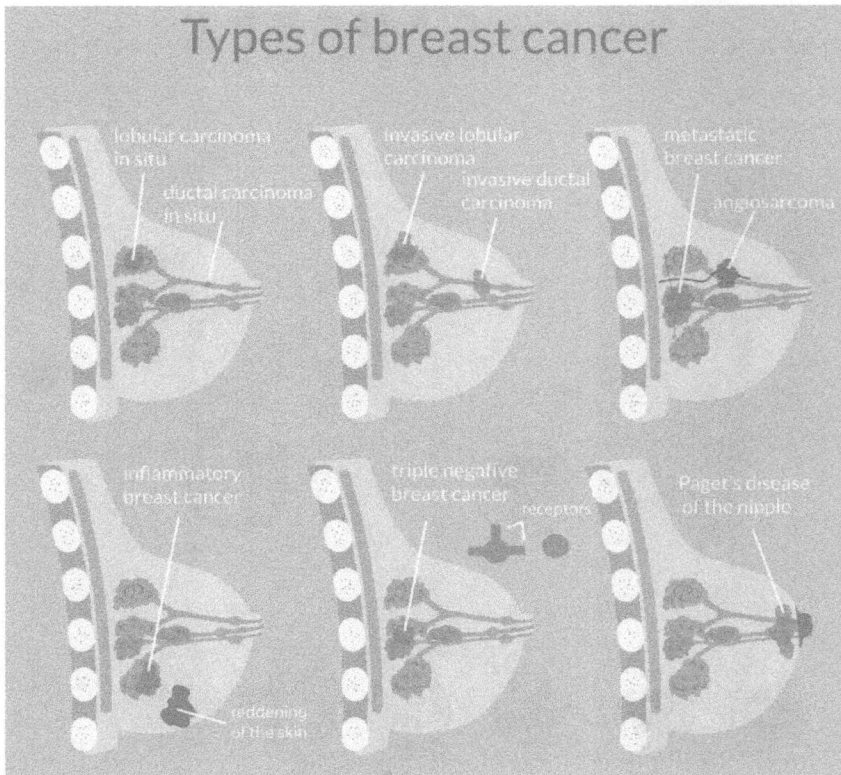

Figure 27

Lobular Neoplasia

This is when there are abnormal cells in the lobules. This is not as common as ductal carcinoma. The types of lobular abnormalities are divided into the following:

- Atypical lobular hyperplasia (ALH): A portion of women with ALH go on to develop cancer in the same breast or the opposite breast.
- Lobular carcinoma in situ (LCIS): Changes have happened in the lobules but not in the nearby tissue, increased risk of having cancer in both breasts.

- Pleomorphic lobular cells in situ (PLCIS): An aggressive variation of lobular carcinoma in situ.

The above are abnormal conditions that require close follow up after treatment of the initial lesion. Medication to prevent recurrence or progression (chemoprevention) may be recommended for a period of time after the diagnosis. This may include medication such as tamoxifen, raloxifene, or other newer agents. Some ladies may even decide to remove the breasts completely, depending on their family history and the presence of other risk factors.

Special Types of Breast Cancer

There are many special types of breast cancer. Please find below a brief summary of some of the more common subtypes.

Inflammatory Breast Cancer

Inflammatory breast cancer is a rare type of invasive breast cancer that accounts for a small percentage of cancers (1-5%). It tends to be more aggressive than other types. It often presents in younger women, obese women, or black women. The symptoms include a red, itchy breast, swelling, skin changes, and nipple retraction. Inflammatory breast cancer usually does not present with a lump in the breast. This makes it harder to diagnose because a mammogram might not detect it. When inflammatory breast cancer is diagnosed, it may have already metastasized and is more likely to be at an advanced stage of disease. This cancer is diagnosed with a biopsy like other cancers.

Paget's Disease of the Nipple

Paget's disease is uncommon, accounting for only about 1-3% of all cases of breast cancer. It presents as a pink or red scaly patch or plaque that starts in the breast ducts and moves to the skin of the nipple and then to the areola (the dark circle around the nipple). You may have symptoms such as nipple discharge, nipple retraction, pruritus, and a breast mass. A palpable breast mass is present in one third of patients.

Paget's disease of the nipple can be confused with atopic dermatitis or eczema. A breast biopsy will help to confirm the diagnosis by showing Paget cells on histology. If you have biopsy-confirmed Paget's disease of the nipple, you should have a mammogram to evaluate for underlying breast cancer. Sometimes the disease also presents with other forms of breast cancer.

Mammography may be helpful, but it can also miss the presence of disease or underestimate the extent of the disease. Therefore, biopsy is indicated for nipple lesions if Paget's disease is clinically suspected, even with normal mammographic findings. Breast magnetic resonance imaging (MRI) may also be useful to help evaluate the extent of disease. Prognosis depends on the stage of the disease and tumor characteristics. The survival rate for patients with Paget's disease is favorable. But if you have had a nipple lesion that has healed you should bring it to your health care provider's attention.

Angiosarcoma
Sarcomas of the breast are rare and make up less than 1% of all breast cancers that start in the cells that line the blood vessels or lymph vessels. This type of breast cancer is divided into primary and secondary cancers and can involve the breast tissue or the breast skin. Primary cases have no preceding cause. Secondary cases may be related to prior radiation therapy in that area. The mass may present with easy bruising in the breast or a lump.

Mammary Adenoid Cystic Carcinoma
Mammary adenoid cystic carcinoma (ACC) is a rare subtype of breast cancer with a favorable prognosis, though it has different

subtypes within it that may be more aggressive. It usually presents as a painful mass that tends not to spread (metastasize) to the lymph nodes.

Breast Metastasis
Other parts of the body that a cancer may metastasize to or spread to include the skin (melanoma), stomach, pancreas, brain, lungs, womb, bones, liver, and thyroid. Imaging may show one lesion or more than one lesion. Sometimes, no lesion is seen on imaging at all. Special studies of breast tissue samples may be helpful in determining whether a lesion started in the breast or in another part of the body. Metastasis may be responsible for pain in a patient, which is important to deal with.

Lymphoma
Lymphoma can start in the breast (primary) or it can be a secondary site of the disease (secondary). Both types of breast lymphoma are rare. These tumors tend to be large (e.g., 4–5 centimeters) compared to typical breast cancer tumors and they tend to look different on imaging due of a lack of calcification. B-cell non-Hodgkin's lymphoma is the most common type. This is when the B cells increase in an abnormal way. Treatment usually includes removing the area of concern and then following surgery with chemotherapy or radiation.

Breast Implant-Associated Anaplastic Large Cell Lymphoma
Breast implant associated-anaplastic large cell lymphoma (BIA-ALCL) is a rare type of cancer that causes tumors in the hematopoietic and lymphoid tissue. BIA-ALCL may start from a pre-existing lymphoproliferative disorder (LPD). It is characterized by an indolent (lazy, slow growing, non-aggressive) localized (in situ) disease in the majority of reported cases. In many cases, it is cured by capsulectomy and implant removal.

Plasmacytoma

Plasmacytoma may or may not cause a lump in the breast. Sometimes Plasmacytoma is associated with a disorder called multiple myeloma. The appearance of this lesion may vary from a single discrete lesion to multiples diffused lesions. A core biopsy is needed to make a diagnosis, along with close inspection under a microscope to look for plasma cells. In this case, special tests are also available to confirm the presence of these types of cells. Treatment may require radiation directed at the area. If the disease in the breast is a secondary manifestation of the illness, the treatment of the primary issue would be sufficient to treat the breast.

Subtypes of Breast Cancer

Breast Receptors

Breast cancer can make receptors in its cells that are designed to respond to specific hormones, such as estrogen, progesterone, or HER2/ERBB2. Think of a receptor and the substance that sticks to it like a lock and key. The receptor is the lock and the substance it binds to it is the key.

If these receptors are present, you can use medications designed to fight them as part of your treatment plan. If your breast cancer does not have estrogen, progesterone, or ERBB2 (formerly called HER2/neu) receptors, it is called triple negative breast cancer. Triple negative breast cancer usually has a less favorable prognosis and is more likely to recur (come back after treatment).

There are five main intrinsic or molecular subtypes of breast cancer that are based on the genes a cancer expresses. Some tumors will express the receptors (binding sites for estrogen, progesterone, and HER2) and some won't. The tumors are also evaluated based on the levels of Ki-67, a protein that affects how fast the cancer cells grow.

The five subtypes are:

- Luminal A
- Luminal B
- Triple-negative/basal-like (estrogen/progesterone/HER2 receptor negative)
- HER2-enriched (estrogen and progesterone negative)
- Normal-like

Luminal A breast cancers are low-grade and usually grow slowly. This type of cancer has hormone-receptors (meaning it's positive for estrogen and/or progesterone receptors). It is HER2 negative. Luminal A cancers have the best prognosis of the molecular subtypes.

Luminal B breast cancers tend to grow a bit faster than luminal A, and their prognosis is slightly worse. Luminal B cancers are estrogen-receptor and/or progesterone-receptor positive. They can be either HER2 positive or HER2 negative and have high levels of Ki-67.

Triple-negative/basal-like cancer is more aggressive that luminal A or luminal B cancer. It is more common in women with BRCA1 gene mutations, as well as women of African descent and younger women. This breast cancer does not have hormone receptors (it is estrogen-receptor, progesterone-receptor, and HER2 negative).

HER2-enriched cancers tend to grow faster than luminal cancers and may have a worse prognosis. They are estrogen-receptor and progesterone-receptor negative and HER2 positive. HER2-enriched cancers are a challenge but they can sometimes be treated with therapies that target the HER2 protein.

Normal-like breast cancer is similar to luminal A cancer. It has a better prognosis than Luminal B, triple negative, or HER2 enriched, but a worse prognosis than luminal A . Normal-like cancers are estrogen-receptor and/or progesterone-receptor positive, HER2 negative, and have low levels of the protein Ki-67.

Table 12

Cancer Type	Characteristics	Prognosis
Luminal A	Positive for estrogen-receptors and/or progesterone-receptors. HER2 negative.	Best
Luminal B	Positive for estrogen-receptors and/or progesterone-receptors. Either HER2 positive negative with high levels of Ki-67.	Not good
Triple-negative	Does not have hormone-receptors (estrogen-receptor, progesterone-receptor, and HER2 negative).	Worse
HER2-enriched	Does not have hormone-receptors (estrogen-receptor, progesterone-receptor negative) and HER2 positive.	Worse
Normal-like	Positive for estrogen-receptors and/or progesterone-receptors), HER2 negative, and low levels of Ki-67.	Good

Treatment
Treatment is when you receive a procedure or medication to attempt to remove or slow down the disease process. The treatment will depend on the extent of the disease and your health status. Treatment may be divided into localized treatment and systemic treatment.

Removal of the Lesion
This may involve removal of the lesion alone (called a lumpectomy) or the removal of the entire breast and the lymph nodes.

Local or Systemic Treatment
After removal of the lesion, your doctors, in collaboration with other specialists, will make recommendations for additional treatment. This may be necessary to help you become or remain disease-free.

Chemotherapy
This uses different medications (primarily delivered via the blood vessels) to kill any abnormal cells that may be in the blood stream. It may be given prior to a surgical procedure, after a surgical procedure, or instead of a surgical procedure.

Radiation
This therapy uses energy to shrink tumors prior to surgery, or to kill any remaining abnormal cells in the breast or under the armpit. Radiation may have short- and long-term effects, but these would be reviewed with you by your physician prior to starting treatment

Immunotherapy
Immunotherapy treatments use your immune (defense) system to help kill cancer cells. There are some approved immunotherapy options for patients with tumors that overexpress certain protein receptors. These include the use of targeted antibodies and immune modulators.

Targeted antibodies
These target the pathway of HER2-, estrogen-, and/or progesterone-receptors and may be used to deliver medication that can kill the malignancy. Your oncologist would let you know if you would benefit from the use of this type of medication.

Immunomodulators
These work with the immune system to stop the cancer cells from exploiting (avoiding detection) the immune system's mechanisms. They can also act as a checkpoint by preventing the white blood cells from removing healthy tissue and instead directing them to remove abnormal cells.

Gene Therapy
These tactics are directed at removing, restoring, or increasing the ability of tumor-preventing genes. Additional functions include transferring drug-resistant genes into normal cells to provide chemoprotection during high dose cancer treatment. Genes can also be used to modify the body's immune response to malignancy.

Staging of Breast Cancer
Staging is a term used to describe the extent of the breast cancer disease process. The clinician uses the information gained from the clinical exam, the imaging, and the tissue obtained to determine the severity of the cancer and the parts of the body that are involved. They use the following characteristics:

- Tumor (T) including the size, the presence of receptors, and tumor type.
- Lymph nodes (N) presence, number, and which lymph nodes do or do not contain cancer.
- Metastasis (M) the presence of the tumor in other parts of the body.

All these characteristics are combined and considered in order to determine the stage of the breast cancer. The details of these characteristics are also changed and updated from time to time by expert panels.

Tumor (T)

In the TNM system, the "T" plus a letter or number (0 to 4) is used to describe the size and location of the tumor.

- Tumor size can be measured in either centimeters (cm) or millimeters (mm). A centimeter is close to the width of a regular pencil.

Stage may also be divided into smaller groups that help describe the tumor in more detail. Specific tumor stage information in listed below.

TX: The primary tumor cannot be evaluated.

T0 (T plus zero): There is no evidence of cancer in the breast.

Tis: This is carcinoma in situ. The cancer is confined within the ducts of the breast tissue and has not spread into the surrounding tissue of the breast. There are two types of breast carcinoma in situ:

- **Tis (DCIS):** DCIS is a noninvasive cancer that has not spread past the duct layer where it began.
- **Tis (Paget's):** Paget's disease of the nipple is a rare form of early, noninvasive cancer that is only in the skin cells of the nipple. Sometimes Paget's disease is associated with another invasive breast cancer. If there is another invasive breast cancer, it is classified according to the stage of the invasive tumor.

T1: The tumor in the breast is 20 millimeters (mm) or smaller in size at its widest area. This is close to width of two pencils. This stage is then broken into 4 substages depending on the size of the tumor:

- T1mi is a tumor that is 1 mm or smaller
- T1a is a tumor that is larger than 1 mm but 5 mm or smaller
- T1b is a tumor that is larger than 5 mm but 10 mm or smaller
- T1c is a tumor that is larger than 10 mm but 20 mm or smaller

T2: The tumor is larger than 20 mm but not larger than 50 mm.

T3: The tumor is larger than 50 mm.

T4: The tumor falls into one of the following groups:

- T4a means the tumor has grown into the chest wall.
- T4b is when the tumor has grown into the skin.
- T4c is cancer that has grown into the chest wall and the skin.
- T4d is inflammatory breast cancer.

Node (N)

The "N" in the TNM staging system stands for lymph nodes (see chapter on anatomy). Regional lymph nodes include:

- Axillary lymph nodes (under the arm)
- Above and below the collarbone
- Internal mammary lymph nodes (under the breastbone)

Lymph nodes in other parts of the body are called distant lymph nodes. If the doctor evaluates the lymph nodes before surgery, based on other tests and/or a physical examination, a letter "c" for "clinical" staging is placed in front of the "N." If the doctor evaluates the lymph nodes after surgery (a more accurate assessment) a letter "p" for "pathologic" staging is placed in front of the "N." The information below describes the pathologic staging.

NX: The lymph nodes were not evaluated.

N0: Either of the following is the case:

- No cancer was found in the lymph nodes.
- Only areas of cancer smaller than 0.2 mm are in the lymph nodes.

N1: The cancer has spread to 1-3 axillary lymph nodes and/or the internal mammary lymph nodes. If the cancer in the lymph node is larger than 0.2 mm but 2 mm or smaller, is it called "micrometastatic" (N1mi).

N2: The cancer has spread to 4-9 axillary lymph nodes, or it has spread to the internal mammary lymph nodes, but not the axillary lymph nodes.

N3: The cancer has spread to 10 or more axillary lymph nodes, or it has spread to the lymph nodes located under the clavicle, collarbone, over the clavicle (supraclavicular), or the internal mammary lymph nodes.

Metastasis (M)
The "M" in the TNM system represents whether the cancer has spread to other parts of the body, called distant metastasis.

MX: Distant spread cannot be evaluated.

M0: The disease has not metastasized.

M0(i+): There is no clinical or radiographic evidence of distant metastases. Microscopic evidence of tumor cells are found in the blood, bone marrow, or other lymph nodes, which are no larger than 0.2 mm.

M1: There is evidence of metastasis to another part of the body, meaning there are breast cancer cells growing in other organs.

Once the TNM characteristics about a breast cancer have been obtained they can be used to determine the staging. The staging takes into consideration the whole picture. It is beneficial for you to be familiar with your stage of disease, if you are diagnosed with breast cancer.

Stage 0: The disease is only in the ducts of the breast tissue (non-invasive). It has not spread to the surrounding tissue of the breast (Tis, N0, M0).

Stage IA: The tumor is small, invasive, and has not spread to the lymph nodes (T1, N0, M0).

Stage IB: Cancer has spread to the lymph nodes and the cancer in the lymph nodes is larger than 0.2 mm but less than 2 mm in size. There is either no evidence of a tumor in the breast or the tumor in the breast is 20 mm or smaller (T0 or T1, N1, M0).

Stage IIA: Any of the following conditions:

- There is no evidence of a tumor in the breast, but the cancer has spread to 1-3 axillary lymph nodes. It has not spread to distant parts of the body (T0, N1, M0).
- The tumor is 20 mm or smaller and has spread to the axillary lymph nodes (T1, N1, M0).

- The tumor is larger than 20 mm but not larger than 50 mm and has not spread to the axillary lymph nodes (T2, N0, M0).

Stage IIB: Either of these conditions:

- The tumor is larger than 20 mm but not larger than 50 mm and has spread to 1-3 axillary lymph nodes (T2, N1, M0).
- The tumor is larger than 50 mm but has not spread to the axillary lymph nodes (T3, N0, M0).

Stage IIIA: The cancer of any size has spread to 4-9 axillary lymph nodes or to internal mammary lymph nodes. It has not spread to other parts of the body (T0, T1, T2 or T3, N2, M0). Stage IIIA may also be a tumor larger than 50 mm that has spread to 1-3 axillary lymph nodes (T3, N1, M0).

Stage IIIB: The tumor has spread to the chest wall or caused swelling or ulceration of the breast or is diagnosed as inflammatory. It may or may not have spread to up to 9 axillary or internal mammary lymph nodes. It has not spread to other parts of the body (T4; N0, N1 or N2; M0).

Stage IIIC: A tumor of any size that has spread to 10 or more axillary lymph nodes, the internal mammary lymph nodes, and/or the lymph nodes under the collarbone. It has not spread to other parts of the body (any T, N3, M0).

Stage IV (metastatic): The tumor can be any size and has spread to other organs, such as the bones, lungs, brain, liver, distant lymph nodes, or chest wall (any T, any N, M1).

Stages of Breast Cancer

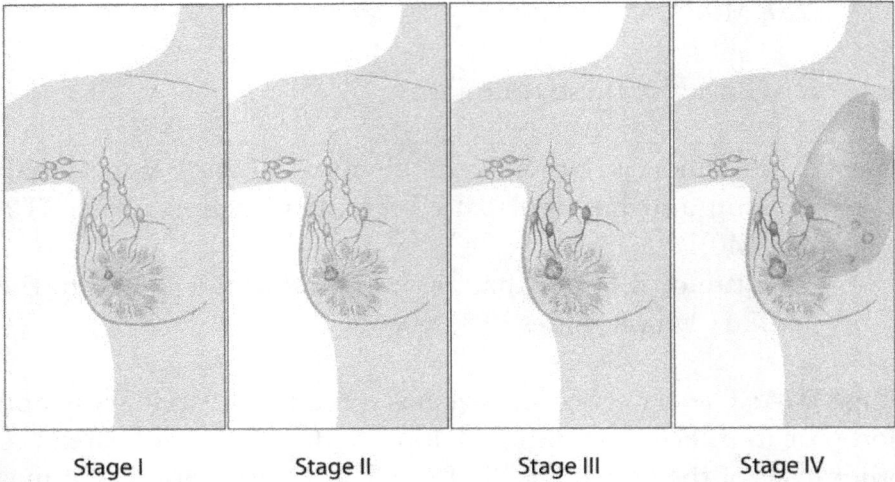

| Stage I | Stage II | Stage III | Stage IV |

Figure 28

Recurrent: Recurrent cancer is cancer that has come back after treatment. It may be described as in the organ (local), in the area (regional), and/or in other parts of the body (distant). If the cancer does return, additional imaging and testing may be done to determine the extent of the recurrence.

Concluding Thoughts on Breast Cancer
Cancer is a not an easy diagnosis to bear. But it is important to keep your hope in place. Treatment is changing as new information becomes available. I suggest that you seek recent, up-to-date sources of information, including talking with your health care provider. Find out your options and do your own research as well. You are an important advocate for yourself in your own care.

Prayer and Meditation

Meditation

Meditation is when you use mindfulness and focus to be able to direct your attention and awareness. It has been shown to help decrease fatigue and stress levels.

Prayer

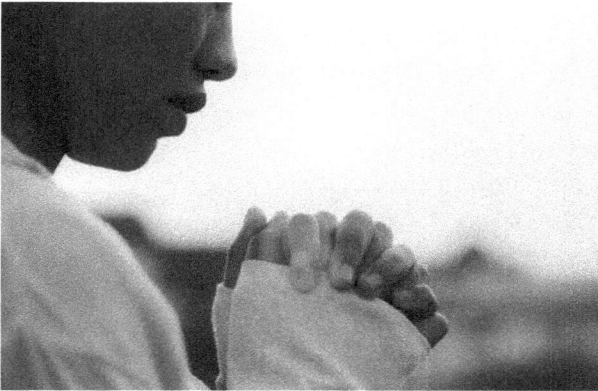

Figure 29 Lady in Prayer

Prayer is communication. It is a request to a deity. In Christianity, this deity is God. It is an act of worship. Studies have shown that prayer has a positive role in helping breast cancer patients cope with diagnosis and treatment processes.

Scriptures of Encouragement

2 Thessalonians 3:16 (NIV)

"Now may the Lord of peace himself give you peace at all times and in every way. The Lord be with all of you."

Luke 8:50 (NIV)

"Hearing this, Jesus said to Jairus, 'Don't be afraid; just believe, and she will be healed.'"

Psalm 34:19 (NIV)

"The righteous person may have many troubles, but the Lord delivers him from them all."

Isaiah 38:16-17 (NIV)

"Lord, by such things people live; and my spirit finds life in them too. You restored me to health and let me live. Surely it was for my benefit that I suffered such anguish. In your love you kept me from the pit of destruction; you have put all my sins behind your back."

Psalm 33:20-22 (KJV)

Our soul waiteth for the Lord: he is our help and our shield.

For our heart shall rejoice in him, because we have trusted in his holy name.

Let thy mercy, O Lord, be upon us, according as we hope in thee.

Philippians 4:6-7 (NIV)

Do not be anxious about anything, but in every situation, by prayer and petition, with thanksgiving, present your requests to God. And the peace of God, which transcends all understanding, will guard your hearts and your minds in Christ Jesus.

Summary Points

- Breast cancer is when breast cells grow abnormally.
- Breast cancer may have different symptoms at presentation.
- Breast cancer may be confined to the area that it starts in, or it may move to other areas.

- Breast cancer type is determined through testing a tissue sample.
- Breast cancer is classified based on the type of receptors that are present.
- Breast cancer treatment is changing as new information is becoming available.
- If you or a loved one have been diagnosed with breast cancer, it is important to be encouraged.
- You should seek treatment and support during this time.
- Do not take this journey alone.

CHAPTER 17

DIAGNOSTIC AND THERAPEUTIC BREAST PROCEDURES

❧

Isaiah 41:10 (NIV)

So do not fear, for I am with you;
do not be dismayed, for I am your God.
I will strengthen you and help you;
I will uphold you with my righteous right hand.

In the following paragraphs I will outline some of the most common diagnostic procedures that may be used to diagnose and/or treat conditions of the breast. Some of these procedures may feel anxiety provoking, but knowing what is involved can help decrease that feeling. Procedures are grouped into two main categories:

- Diagnostic procedures help determine what the problem is
- Therapeutic procedures help treat the problem

Diagnostic Procedures
Needle localization procedures are useful in trying to diagnose breast cancer and breast abnormalities. Biopsies can be done with the help of ultrasound to determine the location of breast lesions.

Fine Need Aspiration (FNA)
This is performed with a small needle that is used to sample cells which are then evaluated under a microscope. This procedure usually only takes a few minutes to perform. Sometimes local pain medication is used and sometimes it is not needed.

Ultrasound-Guided Biopsy
This is when an ultrasound is used to help perform either a fine needle aspiration or a core biopsy. In an ultrasound-guided procedure, the probe is advanced posterior to the lesion. The practitioner will use the imaging to guide them in taking the sample. Think of it as having a way to see the area that you are interested in sampling. As a result, the physician is better able to test the correct area.

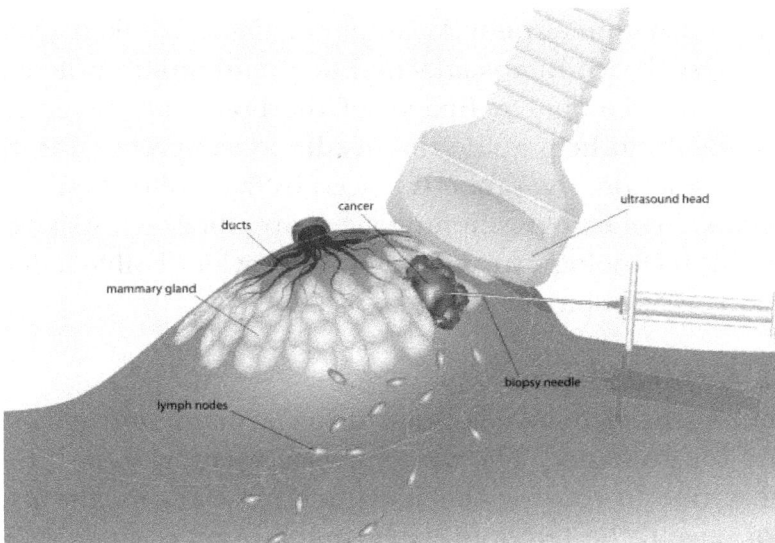

Figure 30 Picture of Ultrasound-Guided Biopsy

Large Core Biopsy
These biopsies use a larger needle than the one used for fine needle aspiration in order to retrieve a larger amount of tissue. You may have one of the following types of biopsy:

- Core biopsy
- Stereotactic core biopsy
- Vacuum-assisted biopsy

Core Biopsy
A core biopsy uses a hollow needle to take a sample of breast tissue This is performed by a biopsy gun. A core biopsy allows removal of a larger specimen than fine needle aspiration. It is more invasive, but it has a better chance of giving a tissues diagnosis. Several tissue samples may be taken at the same time. The sample will be sent to a laboratory to be examined under a microscope.

Stereotactic Core Biopsy
This type of biopsy is used when the area of concern can only be seen on a mammogram. A sample of tissue is taken using a needle biopsy device that is attached to a mammogram machine and linked to a computer. Images of the breast are taken from different angles to help guide the needle to the precise location. To target the lesion, the probe is placed in front of or behind the lesion and stereotactic positioning views are obtained. As a result of using this technology, your health care provider is able to locate and adequately sample the correct area.

Vacuum-Assisted Biopsy
A vacuum-assisted biopsy is done using a mammogram or ultrasound for guidance. The device uses a vacuum to pull tissue into the probe to retrieve the specimen. As a result, the probe does not have to be removed each time a sample is taken. This can be combined with stereotactic biopsy or ultrasound-guided

biopsy to achieve the best results. Multiple samples are obtained using the probe in order to get enough tissue to make a reliable diagnosis.

If post-biopsy images reveal that the lesion has been removed, a percutaneous clip is placed to mark the biopsy site for follow-up examination and possible further treatment. Your healthcare provider will give you follow-up instructions and may ask to see you again to assess for any possible issues such as discomfort, bruising, or swelling at the biopsy site.

Ductoscopy
In this procedure, a small fiberoptic camera is placed in the opening of the breast to look at the ductal system. This test may be recommended if you are having breast discharge.

Therapeutic Breast Procedures
Therapeutic breast procedures use the clinician's expertise to treat a problem. The therapy goal is to readdress the cancer and enable your body to be healed/restored to a disease-free state.

Breast Lumpectomy
This is a surgical procedure wherein the cancerous area of the breast and some nearby normal tissue are removed. A lumpectomy has the best chance of maintaining the breast shape and size and is one of the most common surgical treatments for breast cancer. This procedure is a breast conserving surgery (BCS).

This approach is sufficient for many breast cancers. Once removed, a pathologist evaluates the area of normal tissue that was surrounding the abnormal area (margins) to make sure that all of the abnormal tissue was removed. If all of the abnormal tissue was not removed, a second procedure may be required to remove the rest. Later, additional treatment may be administered to the remaining breast tissue in order to minimize the chance of the cancer returning (recurrence).

Mastectomy
This is an operation that removes most of the breast tissue, except for the chest muscles (pectoralis muscles). This is used for extensive tumors or for patients who do not want a lumpectomy. In some cases, one breast is removed and in other cases, both breasts are removed (bilateral mastectomy). The goal of this procedure is to remove the affected breast tissue in order to prevent a local recurrence of the cancer. The main types of mastectomy performed are:

- Total mastectomy (TM): Involves removal of the breast and removal of the overlying skin. Reconstruction is not required with this procedure.
- Skin-sparing mastectomy (SSM): Involves sparing the skin of the breast but removing the nipple and areola. This type of procedure requires breast reconstruction.
- Nipple-sparing mastectomy (NSM): This involves sparing the skin, areola, and nipple. If the nipple is able to be preserved, this assists with reconstruction. This procedure also requires breast reconstruction. There are many different types of breast reconstruction, including breast implants and muscle transfer flaps. The reconstruction may be done at the time of the initial procedure or it may be done at a later date.

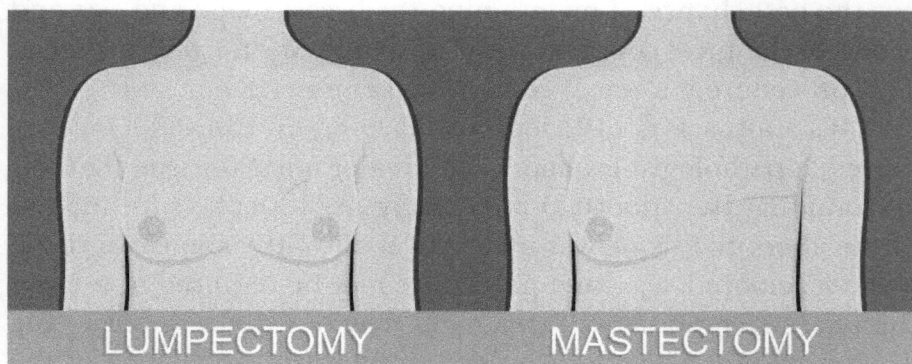

Figure 31 Breast Procedures

Sentinel Lymph Node Biopsy

This is a surgical technique used to identify which lymph nodes drain the area of a breast cancer. A blue dye or radioactive tracer is injected into the tumor, nipple, or area around the tumor before surgery. They then use the dye to find the lymph nodes that the dye drains into. The first lymph node is called the sentinel lymph node. Once removed (excised), the lymph nodes are tested to see if they are involved in the breast cancer. In some situations, sentinel lymph node removal is adequate and axillary lymph node dissection is not needed.

Axillary Lymph Node Dissection

If indicated, some lymph glands under the arm are removed. The lymph nodes are divided into different levels and are removed when deemed surgically necessary.

Summary Points

- A therapeutic procedure is designed to treat the disease process.
- A lumpectomy is removal of the abnormal area along with some normal tissue.
- A mastectomy is removal of the entire breast. It can be unilateral or bilateral.
- A sentinel node biopsy is removal of the lymph nodes involved in the cancer.
- Axillary lymph node dissection is removal of lymph nodes that drain the breast.

CHAPTER 18
PLASTIC AND COSMETIC SURGERY
OF THE BREASTS

❧

Psalm 139:14 (ESV)

I praise you, for I am fearfully and wonderfully made.
Wonderful are your works; my soul knows it very well.

Song of Solomon 8:8 (KJV)

We have a little sister, and she hath no breasts: what shall we
do for our sister in the day when she shall be spoken for?

God has given you your body to manage and your decision to have any surgery should be approached with diligence and care. This decision is yours to make. You should be aware that the effects of surgery are far reaching and long term (if not permanent). In the following section, we will discuss cosmetic and plastic surgery. We will also review how to select a doctor. We will take a look at some of the common breast procedures, including their associated complications.

Plastic Surgery
Plastic surgery is a surgical specialty that involves restoration, reconstruction, and changes to the human body. Plastic surgery on the breasts may be done for different reasons, such as reconstruction after breast cancer or reconstruction due to other breast issues.

Cosmetic Surgery
This entails surgery on a body part for the sole purpose of improving the way it looks.

Selecting a Surgeon
Whether you have a cosmetic or plastic surgeon will depend on your preference. Discuss any procedures that you are thinking about having with your obstetrician/gynecologist. They can offer advice about having a procedure in terms of your fertility and other plans. For example, I have had patients who had an abdominoplasty (tummy tuck) before they had completed childbearing. As a result, they required a cesarean delivery.

A good rule of thumb is to take the time to do your research. You care about the way that you look and want the best outcome possible. I suggest taking the time to have a consultation so that you can express your expectations and see if the surgeon is able to help you achieve these goals. You may want to review the surgeon's portfolio or previous cases. You should check that they have training in the procedure that you are looking to have done. If you have a special type of skin, you may benefit from a surgeon who is used to operating on your skin type.

There are many resources available to help you know what to look for in a surgeon, including the American Board of Cosmetic Surgery or the local medical council. They can let you know which physicians have training in this area and are qualified to perform your procedure.

Some Non-Surgical Procedures in Cosmetic and Plastic Surgery for the Breasts Include:

- Fat transfer to the breasts
- Radiotherapies
- Platelet-rich plasma (PRP)

Fat Transfer to the Breasts
This is when liposuction is performed, the fat is removed and treated, and then used to increase the breast size. The breasts may be treated in advance of the procedure to maximize the results. Use of your own fat cells may reduce the need for breast implants. This usually requires several sessions. Information is still being gathered on the safety and effectiveness of this procedure.

Radiofrequency therapies
Radiofrequency is a type of energy designed to heat the skin (epidermis). When the skin is heated, collagen production is thought to increase, resulting in firmer skin and the breasts getting a lift. Sometimes these two modalities are combined.

Platelet Rich Plasma (PRP)
This is a non-surgical method that injects a component of your own blood (platelet-rich plasma) into the breasts to stimulate their growth. It may also be useful in improving the shape and appearance of the breasts, including skin texture, tone, breast volume, fullness, and nipple sensitivity. The blood is taken from your body

and then placed into a machine that separates it into different components. The platelet-rich portion of the blood has also been shown to have an increased level of growth factors that play a key role in healing and encouraging your body to produce new tissue. It may take 4-6 weeks to see changes and one may need to repeat the treatment process in the future. One should note that this procedure is not a replacement for a breast lift. Your surgeon would discuss possible treatment courses with you and whether this is a possible option.

Surgical Procedures in Cosmetic and Plastic Surgery for the Breasts

Surgery is when an operation is performed. There are many surgeries that can be done to the breasts, but some of the main procedures are as follows:

- Breast lift
- Breast augmentation
- Breast reconstruction
- Breast reduction
- Fat transfer to the breasts
- Nipple lift
- Nipple reduction
- Correction of inverted nipples

Breast Lift (Mastopexy)

The breasts are affected by changes in the body, such as pregnancy, weight gain, weight loss, and the natural processes of age and genetics. As a result, the breasts may become saggy, and you may not be pleased with their appearance.

This a procedure that is done to elevate the breasts. It can be done if the nipples are sagging or enlarged or the breasts are dropping. The breasts may have excess tissue and can be reshaped.

There are different types of breast lifts available and your surgeon would recommend which would be best for you based on your desired results. This procedure will not increase the size of the breasts and can be combined with other breast procedures if indicated. This may affect your milk supply if you intend to breastfeed.

Breast Lift Surgery

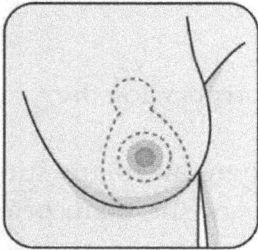

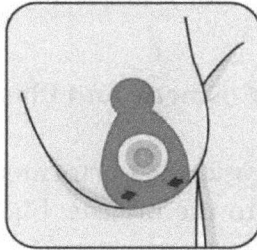

Design phase · Nipple moved up · Skin tightened · Suture

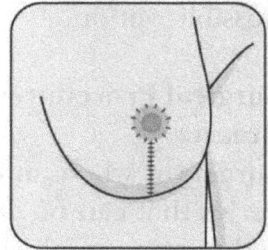

Figure 32 Breast Lift

Breast Augmentation
This is a procedure where the size of the breasts are increased. This procedure uses implants that may be made of different materials to increase the volume, fullness, and/or projection of the breasts.

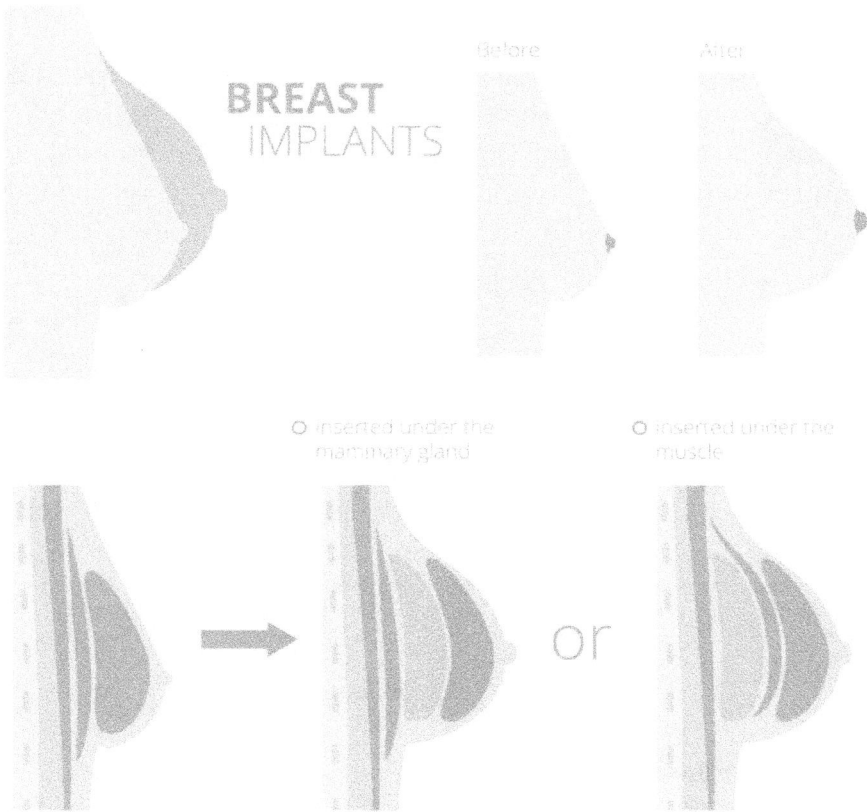

Figure 33 Breast Augmentation Options for Insertion of Implants

An implant is an artificial medical prosthesis that is placed inside the breasts. The main types are made of silicone, saline, or alternative materials. Depending on the material of the implants, they may last about 10 years. Some may last longer, and some may last less.

Surgeons have different techniques for inserting implants, including from underneath the breasts (inframammary), through the nipple, or under the armpits (transaxillary).

Breast Reduction

Breast reductions are also called breast mammaplasty. This is a procedure where the size of the breasts is reduced. It is usually sought if the breasts are causing neck, back, or shoulder pain.

Breast Reduction Surgery

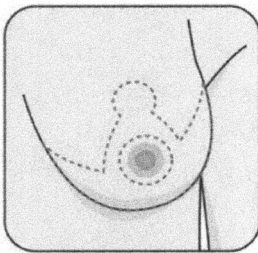

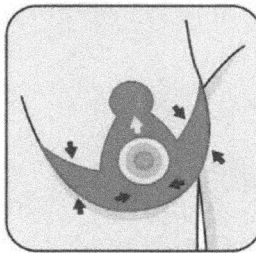

Design phase   • Nipple moved up
                 ● Skin tightened   Suture

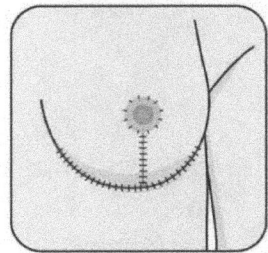

Figure 34 Breast Reduction

Breast Reconstruction

This is when the breast is reformed. Reconstruction can be done when you have a problem with the way the breast was formed or if you have had to have the breast removed for any reason. You and your surgeon will decide which breast reconstruction is the best for you.

Nipple Lift

This is a surgery that is used in people who have finished child-bearing and may have lost volume or elasticity in the breast. This may be done on its own or combined with another procedure such as breast implants. Your surgeon would let you know if this procedure would be beneficial to you.

Nipple Reduction
This is a surgical procedure to reduce the size of the areola tissue. This may be combined with another procedure such as a breast lift or augmentation.

Complications of Breast Surgery
Even though there may be a good reason for the surgery, you must also understand that there are some risks associated with these procedures. Plastic and cosmetic surgery have inherent risks and possible complications, just like any other procedures, such as:

- Seroma
- Blood loss
- Scar tissue
- Hematoma
- Nerve damage
- Clots such as deep vein thrombosis and clots in the lungs called pulmonary embolism
- Anesthesia complications

Seroma: This is a condition where body fluid is built up beneath the surface of the skin and is causing pain. Sometimes these collections will drain out of the body without additional procedures, but sometimes they may need to be drained by your surgeon. They can also get infected and would need to be treated with antibiotics or they may cause swelling and pain. Let your surgeon know if you have any concerns about your incision or if you suspect that this may be happening.

Blood loss: Any procedure has a risk of bleeding since tissue that has blood flowing to it is being cut. If bleeding occurs, it is usually able to be controlled by your surgeon who can use different techniques, instruments, and products to stop it. If the bleeding is significant, sometimes you may need blood or products made from blood to restore your supply and assist in healing.

Scar tissue: Scar tissue can form when normal tissue is impacted by disease, surgery, or injury. It may be a source of skin discoloration or pain. Some people's tissue forms keloids when cut. If you are prone to this, I suggest letting your physician know.

Hematoma: This is a pocket of blood that may be painful and look like a bruise. Many times, a hematoma will be reabsorbed by the body and will clear up with time. Sometimes the hematoma has to be opened and drained. If there is a blood vessel that is bleeding and causing the hematoma, it would need to be stopped.

Infection: Infection happens when the tissue has been contaminated with bacteria. It can cause fever, discoloration of the area, pain, swelling, and/or redness at the incision site. If you think that you have an infection you should let your health care provider know immediately.

Nerve damage or change in skin sensitivity: Nerve damage may happen as the result of surgery. Nerves are responsible for sensation and movement. They run all over your body like highways in a city. In the process of doing surgery, nerves are cut. Sometimes they are injured from a body position or the use of instruments during the procedure. These will often heal with time, but sometimes you may feel a stinging sensation as they are healing. Sometimes they require additional therapy, especially if it is a nerve that impacts motor function. In rare cases, the nerve damage may never improve, leaving you with long-term deficits.

Clots: Clots such as deep vein thrombosis (a clot in the leg) and pulmonary embolism (a clot in the lung) can happen as a result of genetics, having surgery, or being immobile during and after surgery. This may cause no symptoms, shortness of breath, leg swelling, redness in the calf, pain, or death. This is a serious condition that may require medication to thin the blood and prevent future clots. You may also have to have the clot removed or other procedures done. Please let your provider know if you think you have a clot in the leg or the lungs.

Anesthesia

Anesthesia is the medication that is used to ensure your comfort during a surgical procedure. Sometimes you are awake and given medication that only affects the areas that are being operated on, which is called local or regional anesthesia. Sometimes the anesthesia may affect the entire body, which is called general anesthesia. Anesthesia complications may include reactions to the anesthetics, nausea, or vomiting. Some people may also have an allergic reaction to the medication. There are medications available to address these issues.

Your anesthesiologists are experts at handling any issues that may arise. They can explain what can be done about any concerns you may have. You can consult with them before or see them at the time of the procedure.

Number post surgery instruction list

Each procedure will have different instructions before and after, but these are general points to consider:

Read all of the information included in your surgical packet. It may have information that you need to do before, during, and after the procedure. The postoperative course will probably be outlined in this packet. Your physician has taken the time to put together information that they feel is helpful. Use it.

  ✎ Quit smoking prior to any procedure. Smoking interferes with wound healing.

- Discuss how and when you should take any medication that you are given with your doctor or anesthesiologist.
- Take medication as directed for pain.
- If the medication is not working, notify your surgeon.
- If you have a temperature that is greater than 100.4 F, notify your physician.
- If you have drains, record the fluid that drains from the device as directed.
- Follow the directions regarding care of your incisions.
- Wear the recommended support garments.
- Follow the surgeon's instructions.
- Attend all follow-up appointments.

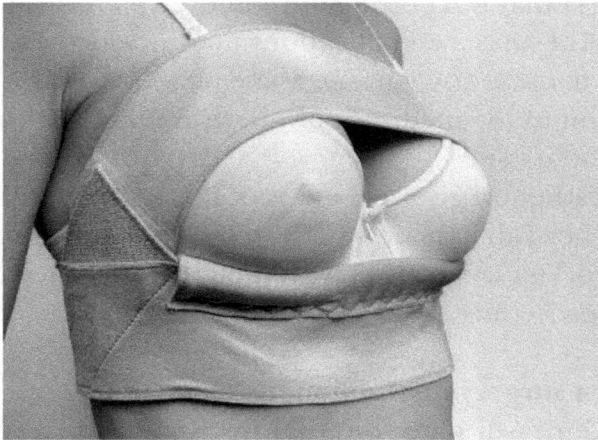

Figure 35 A support garment after plastic surgery

Satisfaction with the Results

Satisfaction is affected by your perception of regular life events and your self-esteem. You may feel shame about your body, which creates stress since your breasts are visible. You may feel good about yourself and want part of you to look different. You could have had something about the way that your breasts where formed that you want to modify or change.

No matter why you are electing to have surgery, make sure that your body is in optimal condition by eating a healthy diet and getting regular exercise prior to any modifications. This will help ensure that you are satisfied with the outcome. It is also important to have reasonable expectations. Take into consideration that your satisfaction and expectations may change with time after you have had your procedure. Sometimes you may continue to be satisfied and sometimes you may have regrets. You should be willing to accept the possibility of both of these emotions.

Romans 14: 12-14 (KJV)
So, then every one of us shall give account of himself to God.
Let us not therefore judge one another anymore: but judge this rather, that no man put a stumbling block or an occasion to fall in his brother's way.
I know, and am persuaded by the Lord Jesus, that there is nothing unclean of itself: but to him that esteemeth anything to be unclean, to him it is unclean.

Consider prayer as part of the process when making a decision to have a surgical procedure.

Cost

Luke 14:28 (NIV)
Suppose one of you wants to build a tower. Won't you first sit down and estimate the cost to see if you have enough money to complete it?

Just like other aspects of healthcare, breast surgery may be costly. When planning and budgeting, take the following into consideration. Costs can include but are noted limited to:

- Anesthesia fees
- Hospital or surgical facility costs

- Medical tests
- Post-surgery garments
- Prescriptions for medication
- Surgeon's fee

If you have insurance, you can check to see if your planned procedure is covered, and if so, what percentage is covered. If you do not have coverage and are paying for the procedure "out of pocket" (with cash), then you can also ask about the cash price. Sometimes discounts are given to people who are paying for surgeries in cash.

Summary Points

- Ensure that your decision has been well thought out.
- Set realistic goals and expectations—down my write them and discuss with your chosen provider.
- Choose a surgeon who has appropriate certifications and experience.
- Understand that some cases have non-surgical and surgical options
- Choose the correct procedure.
- Accept the benefits, risks, and chance of complications associated with the procedure.
- Follow the pre- and post-surgery instructions to achieve the best results.

THE BREASTS AND LIFE'S PHASES

CHAPTER 19

BREAST CHANGES IN PREGNANCY, BREASTFEEDING, AND BEYOND

Psalm 22:9-10 (KJV)

But thou art he that took me out of the womb: thou didst make me hope when I was upon my mother's breasts. I was cast upon thee from the womb: thou art my God from my mother's belly.

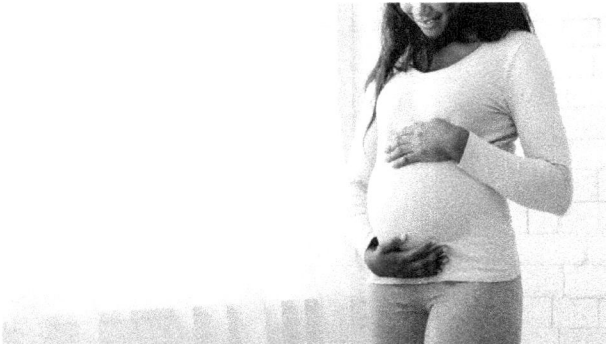

Figure 36 Pregnant Woman

Breast Changes with Pregnancy

The final changes in the breasts happen when you are pregnant. True alveoli appear at this stage. In early pregnancy, you'll have growth and development of the lobule and alveoli. Later in pregnancy, the cells increase in size (hypertrophy) and there are secretions in the alveoli.

In the first trimester, the hormonal changes will often cause breast tenderness. The nipples may also become sensitive or sore and the increased blood flow to the breasts may make them feel heavier. The blood vessels of the breasts may appear more prominent.

In the second trimester, the breast tenderness experienced in the first trimester has usually stopped. The breast tissue grows tremendously in the second trimester. You may even have to purchase a new bra. The milk glands in the breasts (the mammary glands along with the system of ducts that take milk to the nipple) begin to grow in order to ensure a good supply of colostrum (first milk) and continuing milk supply based on your baby's demand after birth. As the blood flow to the breasts increases, you may also notice the veins underneath the skin becoming more visible. Some other changes you may notice include a darkening of the skin around the nipple, known as the areolar, and the appearance of bumps called Montgomery's tubercles. These help to lubricate the nipple with oily secretions to keep it supple and protected as your baby breastfeeds.

In the third trimester the overall weight of the breasts may increase by two to three times and the blood flow doubles. This increase in size may result in stretch marks. In some cases, the breast may also produce milk during the last few weeks of pregnancy.

Breastfeeding

Isaiah 49:15 (NIV)
Can a mother forget the baby at her breast and have no
compassion on the child she has borne? Though she may
forget, I will not forget you!

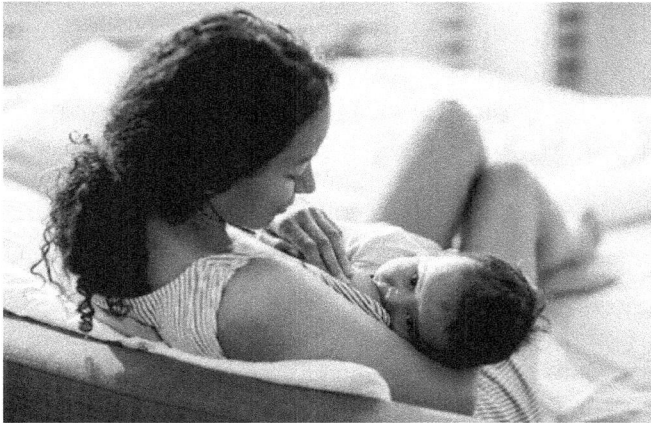

Figure 37 Breastfeeding Mother

Breastfeeding is a way to provide the nutrients that your baby needs while satisfying their hunger and thirst at the same time. It allows for healthy growth and development during the first six months of life. Breastfeeding helps to develop organs such as the jaw, brain, and eyes of your baby. It also helps the baby's body resist infection and disease and reduces the risk of obesity in childhood and adulthood. It is economical, always available, and accessible. Breastfeeding in the immediate postpartum period is also helpful to the mother. It decreases her risk of bleeding in the short-term, and in the long-term, it decreases her risk of breast and ovarian cancer.

Breastfeeding Physiology

Milk supply is controlled by the hormone prolactin. When the infant cries or sucks on the nipple, oxytocin (a hormone) is released in the mother. When oxytocin is released from the pituitary gland, it causes milk release. Milk release is driven by the contraction of the myoepithelial cells around the alveoli and ducts.

Getting Started with Breastfeeding

Many mothers can breastfeed if they choose to. Mothers may produce 600 milliliters of milk or more in a day. Breastfeeding can be challenging, so it is helpful to have support from your family and health care providers. Exclusive breastfeeding is recommended until the baby is six months old in order to maximize the benefits for your infant. Milk production has different stages, which are as follows:

- Colostrum (days 1-2)
- Transitional milk (days 2-5 to up to 2 weeks)
- Mature milk (days 6-15 and beyond)

Colostrum: The is the first milk your breasts make. This milk is clear, creamy, or lemon-yellow in color and quite thick and sticky. It has important substances that help give your baby a great start, such as protein, carbohydrates, antibodies (substances that help fight infection such as IgG, IgM, IgA), and minerals and fat-soluble vitamins (Vitamins A, B, C, and D). It has more protein in the form of globulin and minerals than mature milk. Colostrum lasts for approximately five days and then becomes transitional milk.

Transitional milk: This is the creamy milk that follows colostrum. This milk also has a high protein content.

Mature milk: This milk may be more watery than transitional milk. It comes in by the second week of baby's life. The amount of mature milk may be copious. There are two types: foremilk and hindmilk. The foremilk is what comes out at the start of a feeding session. It has water-soluble vitamins and protein. The hindmilk comes out of the breast towards the end of a feeding session and contains more fat.

How is human milk different from "regular" (animal) milk? Human milk contains all of the vitamins except Vitamin K. It has the same amount of water as animal milk but it contains more carbohydrates and fat and less protein. Human milk is also usually more compatible with the baby's digestive system.

Benefits of breastfeeding to the mother include:

- Helps to prevent postpartum bleeding (hemorrhage)
- Helps your womb return to a normal state
- Helps you to lose weight postpartum
- Keeps your period away, allowing you to increase your red blood count post-delivery
- Acts as a form of contraception (if you are exclusively breastfeeding)
- Reduces risk of osteoporosis in the future
- Decreases risk of cancer of the uterus, ovaries, and breasts
- Saves money
- Makes travelling easier since you have a ready milk supply
- Reduces risk of pneumonia, influenza, urinary tract infections, ear infections, and Haemophilus
- Reduces risk of diabetes, ulcerative colitis, and Chron's disease

Maternal conditions that may affect your breast milk supply:

- Prior breast surgery
- Prior infant conditions, such as low blood sugar or poor infant growth
- Maternal medical conditions
- Maternal breast conditions such as severe asymmetry, tubular breasts, a breast mass. or inverted nipples

Maternal conditions that may affect your ability to breastfeed include:

- HIV that is detectable
- Symptomatic COVID-19

- Infection with human T-cell lymphotropic virus type I or type II
- Untreated active tuberculosis

Positions for Breast Feeding

Different positions may be used to help you and your baby be comfortable during breast feeding and improve your breastfeeding experience. Work with your midwife or lactations consultant to decide which ones are best for you.

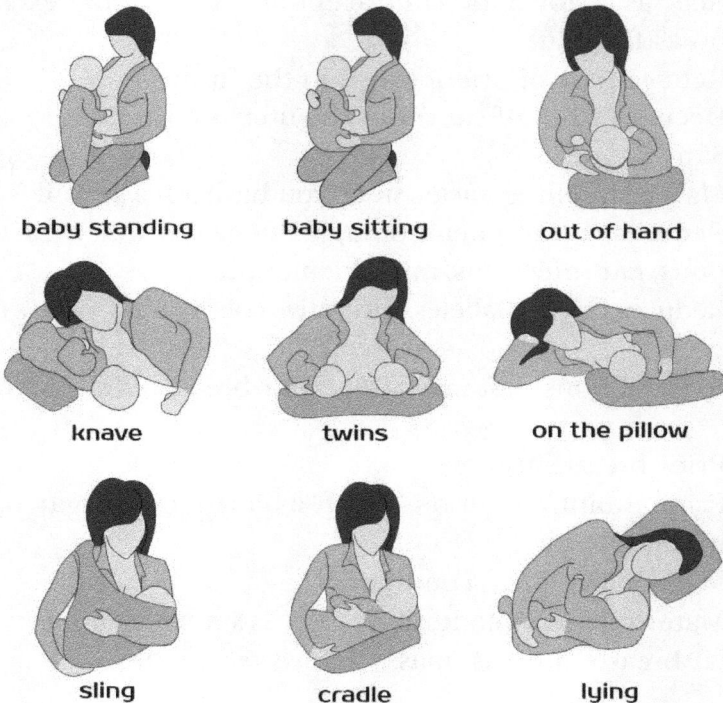

Figure 38 Breast Feeding Positions

Problems with the Breasts While Breastfeeding

Breastfeeding has many benefits to the mother and the infant. When the breast milk first comes in (usually around 3-5 days after delivery) the breasts may feel very full. This fullness may improve with breastfeeding. You may not have any challenges with breast-feeding, but some people do. Even though you might be motivated to breastfeed, you may encounter issues that can be discouraging and painful. These problems include:

- Engorgement
- A blocked duct
- Mastitis
- Large, flat, or inverted nipples
- Cracked nipples/fissures
- Overproduction of milk
- Underproduction of milk

Engorgement
When your milk comes in (called let-down), you may become en-gorged. This usually happens the first 2-4 days after delivery. The breasts become very firm and swollen, which may result in pain and sometimes a mild fever. The expression of the milk ducts near the alveolar region helps to alleviate these symptoms.

An engorged breast may be hard for a baby to latch onto, but be patient and continue trying to breastfeed. Engorgement may be prevented or relieved in the following ways:

- Getting a nursing bra that fits well (see chapter on bra sizing).
- Massaging the breasts manually with your hands to encour-age milk expression.
- Alternating which breast that you offer the baby first.
- Nurse for at least 15-20 minutes on each breast before switching sides to allow for complete emptying of the ducts.
- Adjust the infant's position. Speak with your nurse, midwife or lactation consultant to learn about different breastfeed-ing positions.

- Use a breast pump or older toddler (if tandem nursing) to help relieve a plugged duct.
- Use a heating pad to encourage milk flow or a cooling pad to decrease pain.
- Take a hot shower with the water directed toward the engorged breast.

Blocked duct

This may cause a tender lump in one breast with the skin over the lump appearing red. This is a result of milk not moving from the breast. It can happen if the duct in one part of the breast is blocked by thickened milk, breastfeeding has been infrequent, the infant is latching poorly, or if the breast is being affected by tight clothing or trauma. To deal with this, you would want to identify and remedy the cause of the blocked duct so that the milk could be removed from the breast. In addition to notifying your health care provider, you can also try the following steps:

- Applying warm compresses to the affected breast.
- Varying the position of the baby (across your body or under your arm).
- Feed from the affected breast frequently.
- Gently massaging the breast over the lump while baby is suckling (this can help the thickened milk come out).

Mastitis

This is inflammation and infection of the breast, usually due to a blocked milk duct. (See chapter on mastitis for more information.) If you have mastitis, the affected breast will be red, swollen, and painful, and you may also have a fever and not feel well. This condition is treated with antibiotics and expressing breast milk. Standing under a hot shower can help the milk release. Your baby can also continue to breastfeed to aid in release of the blocked milk duct. Your baby will not get the infection.

Inverted, large, flat, or long nipples

Nipples have different shapes that typically do not affect a mother's ability to breastfeed. But large, flat, or long nipples can make it harder for a baby to latch on. If a flat nipple can be pulled up and out with your fingers (protractile) then you should be able to breastfeed without problems. If the nipple does not stretch and cannot be pull out (non-protractile), the baby may have a hard time breastfeeding. A large or long nipple may make it impossible for a baby to take enough breast tissue into its mouth even when it is opened wide. Tips for this include:

- Trying different breastfeeding positions.
- Allowing the infant to figure out its own method of taking the breast.
- Pumping or expressing milk for the first 1-2 weeks as protractility of the breasts can improve and the size of the baby's mouth will also increase with time.
- Using a syringe that has been modified with your fingers to help adjust the shape of the nipple just before feeding.
- Looking into surgical procedures available for inverted nipples.
- Allowing a lactation consultant to help before delivery or if you encounter difficulty afterward.

Cracked Nipples/Fissures

This is when you have severe nipple pain when the baby is suckling or if there is a visible fissure (crack) across the tip of the nipple or around the base. Poor attachment or incorrect suckling of your infant can cause sore and fissured nipples. If you have a communicable disease like HIV, a crack in the nipple may increase the chance that you can transmit it to your baby. If your baby's position and attachment are improved, this will give the nipple a chance to heal and pain will resolve.

Overproduction of Milk
The mother may have a forceful oxytocin reflex so that her milk flows fast. This can make the baby choke and pull away from the breast during feeds. Your nurse or lactation consultant can check to make sure baby's attachment is adequate. You may try breast-feeding while lying on your back or holding the breast with your fingers closer to the areola during feeds to help control the milk outflow. Another tip is to allow your infant to breastfeed on one breast to empty it at the time of feeding and then use the next breast in the subsequent feed.

Underproduction of Milk
Some mothers have low milk production because of pathological (abnormal) causes, such as endocrine problems (pituitary failure after severe hemorrhage or retained piece of placenta) or poor breast development. If you have low production that does not improve when the breastfeeding technique and pattern are changed, and your exam and the infant is normal, this is called physiological low breast milk production. Smoking and alcohol consumption, severe malnutrition, hormone-containing contraceptive pills, and pregnancy may reduce milk production.

Increasing Your Breast Milk Supply
With proper support and information, most mothers are able to produce more than enough milk for their baby (or babies). However, if you have a low milk supply problem, talk to your health care provider and a lactation expert to evaluate the issue, improve your breastfeeding or expressing technique, or to decide if a galactagogue would be helpful for you.

Galactagogues are substances that cause, increase, or maintain breast milk production. Prolactin is a woman's main breast milk-producing hormone. Most medications that act as galactagogues work by increasing prolactin levels. Galactagogues are foods or medications that may help to increase breast milk supply, such as:

- Oatmeal
- Vitamins (e.g., B-complex)
- Domperidone (Motilium®): A prescription drug used for gastrointestinal disorders
- Chlorpromazine: A prescription drug used as an antipsychotic.
- Sulpiride: An antipsychotic/antidepressant medication that may increase milk production by increasing prolactin
- Metoclopramide (Maxolon®): Another prescription drug used to treat gastrointestinal disorders
- Herbs such as raspberry leaf, nettle, anise, alfalfa, blessed thistle, chaste berry, and fennel
- Fenugreek which is sometimes used as a culinary herb but has historically been used as a galactagogue for both human mothers and dairy animals around the world

The medications mentioned above may increase milk supply, but they can have side effects (especially on the nervous system) such as restlessness, drowsiness, fatigue, and depression. Any usage of the above should be discussed with your health care provider. You can also alternate breastfeeding with bottle-feeding. Some mothers who have to return to work or who have very demanding daily schedules can choose this option. Infants under six months do not need additional water, as mixed formula and breast milk contains enough water for them.

Storage of Milk
Store in small, single-feed quantities of about 2-4 ounces. This prevents wastage of your valuable milk since milk leftover from a feed should be discarded after about an hour. When it is time to use the milk, thaw slowly in the fridge, in a container of cool water, or under

cool running water. Once thawed, you can use it. Do not refreeze thawed milk and never heat breast milk in the microwave or on the stove, as this destroys the protective enzymes and antibodies. If you need to warm the milk, place the bottle or storage bag in a bowl of very warm water. Do not add freshly pumped milk to frozen milk.

Summary Points

- Changes occur in the breasts during and after pregnancy.
- Breastfeeding has many benefits for the mother and the newborn.
- If you decide to breastfeed, set realistic goals and expectations. Be patient with yourself when learning how to breastfeed.
- Get information on correct positioning and how to care for the breasts.
- Breast difficulties may happen, such as engorgement, mastitis, cracked nipples, or under or overabundant milk supply.
- Consider the advice of a lactation consultant if you are not satisfied with your milk supply.
- A galactagogue is a substance that can be used to increase milk supply.

Exodus 2:1-9 (NIV)
Now a man of the tribe of Levi married a Levite woman, and she became pregnant and gave birth to a son. When she saw that he was a fine child, she hid him for three months. But when she could hide him no longer, she got a papyrus basket for him and coated it with tar and pitch. Then she placed the child in it and put it among the reeds along the bank of the Nile. His sister stood at a distance to see what would happen to him.

Then Pharaoh's daughter went down to the Nile to bathe, and her attendants were walking along the riverbank. She saw the basket among the reeds and sent her female slave to get it. She opened it and saw the baby. He was crying, and she felt sorry for him. "This is one of the Hebrew babies," she said.
Then his sister asked Pharaoh's daughter, "Shall I go and get one of the Hebrew women to nurse the baby for you?"
"Yes, go," she answered. So, the girl went and got the baby's mother. Pharaoh's daughter said to her, "Take this baby and nurse him for me, and I will pay you." So, the woman took the baby and nursed him.

CHAPTER 20

CONTRACEPTION AND BREAST HEALTH

❦

Proverbs 5:18-19 (KJV)

Let thy fountain be blessed:
and rejoice with the wife of thy youth.
Let her be as the loving hind and pleasant roe;
let her breasts satisfy thee at all times; and be
thou ravished always with her love.

Contraception is any medication or means that is used to prevent pregnancy. When we talk about contraception, some have concerns about the impact that the medication could have on the breast tissues, especially the risk of breast cancer. Studies have cited "health concerns" as one of the reasons people say they do not want to use contraception. However, there are contraceptive methods that may impact the breasts and others that have no impact on the breasts.

Table 13 Contraceptive Methods—Efficacy, Advantages, Disadvantages, and Breast Impact

Method of contraception	Does it Impact the Breasts? (Yes or No)	Efficacy (%)	Advantages	Disadvantages
Abstinence	No	100	It is free. It protects you from STIs. There are no side effects.	None
Fertility awareness (Rhythm Method)	No	76	Free, no side effects.	You have to have regular cycles to be able to use this method.
Pull out/ withdrawal method (removal of penis before ejaculation)	No	72-96	It is free.	You have to rely on the male partner to participate. It is not as reliable, as sperm can be released before ejaculation.
Spermicide	No	72	It is affordable.	It has to be used correctly. Usage may be a challenge if you have a latex allergy.
Condoms— Male condoms, female condoms	No No	82 79	They are easily accessible, affordable, and easy to carry in a pocket or purse.	They have to be used correctly. Usage may be a challenge if you have a latex allergy. They may break if not used correctly. They do not help with menstrual cycle issues.

(Continued)

Table 13 Contraceptive Methods—Efficacy, Advantages, Disadvantages, and Breast Impact (*Continued*)

Method of contraception	Does it Impact the Breasts? (Yes or No)	Efficacy (%)	Advantages	Disadvantages
Injectables				
Depo-Provera	Yes	91	You do not have to remember to use it daily, so you are less likely to miss an injection. It is reversible; its effects wear off once you stop using it. The effects begin with the first injection. One injection can prevent pregnancy. The side effects may decrease with time.	It may result in irregular bleeding, lack of menses, and weight gain. It may delay ovulation for up to a year after injection. Prolonged use may affect bone mineral density. You may have an increase in breast size.
Mesigyna®	No	94	You use if once a month. You still have a period. It is affordable.	Muscle injection that is given once a month.

(*Continued*)

Table 13 Contraceptive Methods—Efficacy, Advantages, Disadvantages, and Breast Impact (*Continued*)

Method of contraception	Does it Impact the Breasts? (Yes or No)	Efficacy (%)	Advantages	Disadvantages
Noristerat®	No	94	Once every 8 weeks. It is affordable.	Muscle injection. May cause bloating, headache, dizziness, nausea, reaction at the injection site, weight gain, irregular bleeding. Cannot be used if you have porphyria.
Hormonal methods				
Oral contraceptive pill (OCP)	Yes	91–99	It is effective when used as directed. It may improve regularity of cycles. It may decrease pain associated with menses or endometriosis. You are in control and do not need your partner to take this. It decreases the risk of PID (Pelvic Inflammatory Disease). It decreases the risk of endometrial and ovarian cancer.	May cause nausea, vomiting, and breast tenderness in the first 2-3 cycles. Does not protect against STIs. Risk of clots in legs. Check with a physician to ensure that you are able to take them. Oral contraception is not recommended with certain medications or medical problems.

(*Continued*)

Table 13 Contraceptive Methods—Efficacy, Advantages, Disadvantages, and Breast Impact (*Continued*)

Method of contraception	Does it Impact the Breasts? (Yes or No)	Efficacy (%)	Advantages	Disadvantages
Progesterone only pill Low dose High dose	No Yes	92-99	It may decrease bleeding during menses. It does not increase the risk of high blood pressure or heart disease. They can be taken while breastfeeding.	You have to take it every day. You should take it around the same time each day. If you are more than 2-3 hours late, you have to use a backup method for the next 2 days. It may make changes to the menses such as irregular bleeding or spotting between cycles. It is not recommended if you have lupus. It may not work if you are taking HIV, seizure, narcolepsy, or tuberculosis medication. You may have short or heavy cycles, or no period at all. Symptoms such as nausea, headache, and breast tenderness.
Patch	Yes	91	They have easy to follow instructions. They are small.	You must replace it weekly. It may cause skin reactions. It is visible. You may have breast soreness

(*Continued*)

Table 13 Contraceptive Methods—Efficacy, Advantages, Disadvantages, and Breast Impact (*Continued*)

Method of contraception	Does it Impact the Breasts? (Yes or No)	Efficacy (%)	Advantages	Disadvantages
Ring	Yes	91	They are easy to use. You do not need to think about contraception for a month.	Your body may expel it. You may have an increased risk of heart attack and stroke. It is a foreign body.
Emergency contraception (Morning after pill, Plan B, ellaOne)	No	91	It reduces the risk of pregnancy when started.	It may affect your cycle that month.
Implants				
Implantable device (Jadelle®, Implanon®, Nexplanon®)	Yes	99	It is effective when used as directed. It may decrease frequency of periods. It may decrease pain with menses or endometriosis. It is effective for 3-5 years.	You may have breakthrough spotting. You may have pain with menses. An office procedure is required to place and remove it. You may have nipple discharge. You may have breast tenderness or a lump in the breast.

(*Continued*)

Table 13 Contraceptive Methods—Efficacy, Advantages, Disadvantages, and Breast Impact (*Continued*)

Method of contraception	Does it Impact the Breasts? (Yes or No)	Efficacy (%)	Advantages	Disadvantages
Non-hormonal Intrauterine Device (IUD)	No	99.2	It is effective for up to 7 years.	An office procedure is required to place and remove it. Discomfort may be experienced upon placement. It may increase bleeding with menses.
Hormonal Intrauterine Device (IUD)	Yes	99.2	It is effective when used as directed, usually for 3-5 years. It may decrease heaviness and frequency of cycles. It may decrease pain associated with menses or endometriosis.	An office procedure is required to place and remove it. Discomfort may be experienced upon placement. It may decrease bleeding with menses. You may become amenorrhoeic

Contraceptive Methods

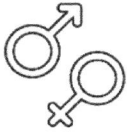

ABSTINENCE

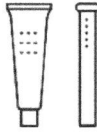

SPERMICIDE

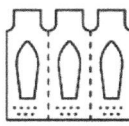

SUPPOSITORIES

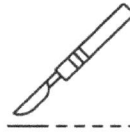

SURGICAL
STERILIZATION

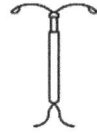

HORMONAL IUD

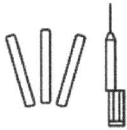

DIAPHRAGM

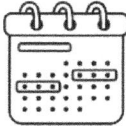

NATURAL FAMILY
PLANNING

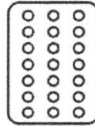

ORAL CONTRACEPTIVES

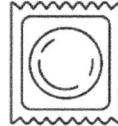

MALE CONDOMS

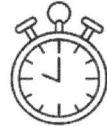

COITUS INTERRUPTUS

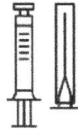

IMPLANT

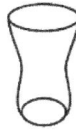

INJECTIONS

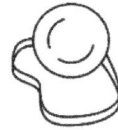

FEMALE CONDOMS

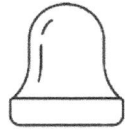

VAGINAL SPONGE

CERVICAL CAP

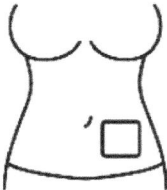

CONTRACEPTIVE PATCH

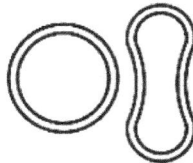

VAGINAL RING

Figure 39 Contraceptive Methods

All the methods used for contraception are outlined above, but the most common methods used by women in the reproductive age group include condoms and birth control pills (with the combined oral contraceptive being the most common type of birth control pill).

Birth control pills have been around for more than 50 years. These are pills that you take every day or for 21 days in a month. They have hormones that prevent pregnancy. There are different types of birth control pills and your doctor can help you pick the one that would best suit you. Sometimes a lady has to try different types before finding the one that best suits her body.

If you have a history of clots in the legs or lungs, a disorder that increases your risk of clots (such as thrombophilia, factor V Leiden mutation, protein C or S deficiency, or antithrombin III), lupus, cyanotic heart disease, or pulmonary artery hypertension, you are not a candidate for the birth control pill. Just like any other medication, the pill has risks and benefits.

Risks may include:

- Clots in the legs and lungs (one in ten thousand ladies)
- Nausea
- Vomiting
- Headache
- Abdominal pain
- Breast tenderness
- Possible increase in breast cancer risk

Benefits may include:

- Decreased bleeding during periods
- Regulation of the period
- Decreased risk of cancers in endometrium
- Decreased risk of ovarian cancer

Hormonal Methods and the Breasts
Some studies have shown an increased risk of breast cancer if you take hormonal contraceptives. Although use of hormonal

contraceptives may increase a person's risk compared to someone who has never used birth control, to put it in perspective, the risk is much less when compared to your risk if you drink alcohol. Ten years after stopping the use of the birth control, the increased risk will go away. Studies have also shown a decreased risk for other types of cancer when taking hormonal contraceptives, such as ovarian, endometrial, and colon. You have to take into consideration all of the possible risks and benefits if you opt to use the birth control pill or other hormonal contraceptives. Your provider will review your family history and possible risks with you to help you make a decision.

Contraceptives for Women with a History of Breast Cancer
Woman who have been treated for breast cancer with tamoxifen should not use hormonal contraceptives. They should use non-hormonal contraception. Those who've had estrogen-receptor-positive breast cancer should take progesterone-only contraception. They can use non-hormonal contraceptives without restriction.

Contraceptives for Women with a Family History of Breast Cancer
Family history of breast cancer in a first degree relative may increase your risk of breast cancer with the use of hormonal methods of contraception. If you have a second- degree relative with a history of breast cancer, it may be preferable to use a low dose formulation of contraception or one without hormones.

Emergency Contraception
This term refers to using contraception to prevent pregnancy within 5 days (120 hours) after unprotected sex. The two main ways to do this are by:

- Using pills designed for this purpose (the morning after pill)
- Inserting a copper intrauterine device (IUD)

Emergency contraception is not meant to be used as your only form of birth control, nor should it be used regularly, as it is not as effective as non-emergency (regular) contraceptive methods. Emergency contraception can be used if you are breastfeeding or if you have breast cancer. After taking emergency contraceptive pills, your period may come earlier or later. If you do not see a period within three weeks after using emergency contraception, you should take a pregnancy test. If the test is negative, you can wait for your period. If it is positive, see your health care provider.

Summary Points

- As an adult, you have to take responsibility for your actions—especially decisions about when to have sex.
- Decide what your goals are for your sexual health.
- If you are sexually active, take the time to review available contraceptive measures and how they may impact breast health.
- Your health care provider will provide a safe, nonthreatening environment for you to discuss your concerns.
- Your health care provider should listen to you and provide you with relevant information.
- Your health care provider will discuss the advantages and disadvantages of your contraceptive options and recommend which one is best for you, especially if you have a breast concern.

CHAPTER 21

BREAST HEALTH, AGING, AND MENOPAUSE

⁓⦿⁓

Isaiah 46:4 (NIV)

*Even to your old age and gray hairs
I am he, I am he who will sustain you.
I have made you and I will carry you;
I will sustain you and I will rescue you.*

Breasts and Aging

The breasts change as we age. Breast development is affected by hormones—specifically estrogen and progesterone. Estrogen regulates the development of the ductal tissue and progesterone regulates the branching of the milk ducts and the development of the lobules. The glandular tissue usually gives breasts their firm or lumpy consistency. As women age, estrogen and progesterone decrease, and androgen hormones increase.

Menopause

The changes that happen in menopause are related to the decrease in estrogen. The lobules and the ducts atrophy. There is an increase in fatty tissue and a decrease in glandular tissue as the glandular parts of the breasts are replaced with fatty tissue. This results in the breasts losing their size or becoming lumpier. The tissue may lose its elasticity and, as a result, the breasts may sag. Some may find that they have breast tenderness or pain as one of their menopausal symptoms. If you experience this, you should discuss it with your health care provider.

Hormone Replacement Therapy (HRT) and Breast Disease

As you enter menopause you may experience symptoms such as hot flashes, irritability, and vaginal dryness. You may wonder what options are available to you to treat these symptoms and the effect that they may have on the breasts.

This is where having a provider who takes care of your entire well-being comes in handy. If you are on HRT for 1-4 years, the risk of breast cancer has not been shown to be any higher. However, once you get into the 5-9-year window, the risk is increased when compared with a lady who has not taken HRT. If a person goes up to 15 years of use, the risk is found to be more than 1.5 times higher than someone who has not taken HRT. This increase in risk decreases when you stop taking the medication. Once you have been off HRT for 5 years or more, there is no longer an increased risk of cancer.

Your health care provider will have a conversation with you and asses your risk in terms of its impact on your breasts and your overall health.

Table 14

National Cancer Institute Risk Assessment		
Risk	**5 year**	**Suggestion**
Low	<1.67	Ok
Intermediate	1.67-5	Proceed with caution
High	>5	Avoid

Several scoring systems are available help calculate your risk with the use of HRT. One system is the National Cancer Institute Risk Assessment. Your provider may use one of the scoring systems along with counselling, and they may discuss alternate measures with you. If you are BRCA positive, it is important to discuss the safety of HRT with your breast oncologist.

Testosterone and DHEA may result in some stimulation of the breast tissue. Your provider may recommend alternatives such as Osphena®, Intrarosa®, or Relizen® for treatment of menopause symptoms. These are not estrogenic, but minimal data exists on their efficacy and safety.

Sagging Breasts
Sagging breasts (known as breast ptosis) are breasts where the tissue is stretched and the nipple and areola hang downward. Although this is more common in menopause, it can happen prematurely in younger women as well. Anything that affects the connective tissue can also weaken the breast tissue and its supports, including:

- Multiple pregnancies. Each pregnancy causes wear and tear on the breasts as it causes them to increase in size while you are pregnant and then decrease in size post-pregnancy or when you stop breastfeeding.
- Larger breasts, as they will be more likely to sag with gravity.

- Chronic illnesses, such as connective tissue disorders or breast cancer.
- Smoking, as the carcinogen negatively impacts the connective tissue in all parts of the body, including the breasts.
- Menopause.
- Weight gain or weight loss.
- Strenuous exercise.

Ptosis (Sagging) Scale

- *Grade I: Mild ptosis:* The nipple is at the level of the inframammary fold and above most of the lower breast tissue.
- *Grade II: Moderate ptosis:* The nipple is located below the inframammary fold but higher than where most of the breast tissue hangs.
- *Grade III: Advanced ptosis:* The nipple is below the inframammary fold and at the level of maximum breast projection.
- *Pseudoptosis:* The nipple is above or at the inframammary fold, but most of the breast tissue is below the level of the fold. This is not considered a true ptosis.
- *Parenchymal Maldistribution:* The lower breast tissue lacks fullness, the inframammary fold is very high, and the nipple and areola are relatively close to the fold.

DEGREES OF PTOSIS

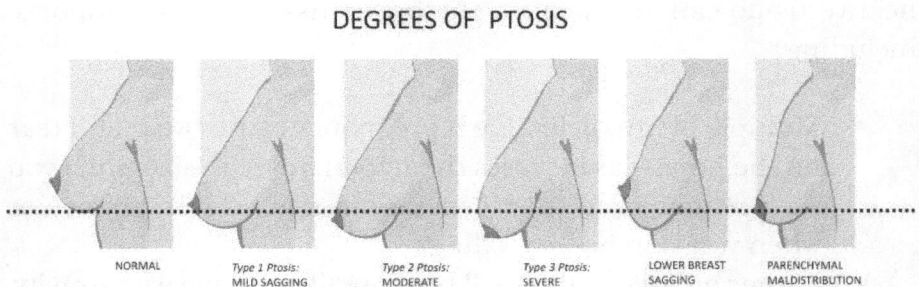

| NORMAL | Type 1 Ptosis: MILD SAGGING | Type 2 Ptosis: MODERATE | Type 3 Ptosis: SEVERE | LOWER BREAST SAGGING | PARENCHYMAL MALDISTRIBUTION |

Figure 40

Measures that help to preserve breast health and delay sagging include:

- Support
- Posture
- Nutrition
- Exercise

Support
Wearing a garment that fits will help lend support to your breasts. This will help to prevent sagging (See chapter on bra fitting). Good support reduces the stress and strain on the breast tissue.

Posture
If your posture is not good, for example if you slouch frequently, this could cause the breasts to appear droopy or sagging. Good posture not only pulls the breasts upward, it also allows the weight to be distributed across the tissues evenly, which is thought to put less strain on the breast tissue.

Nutrition
Eat a healthy and balanced diet to help your skin supple—this will add support to the breasts and delay sagging. If you are overweight, that increases the strain on your tissue, and the extra weight may add additional weight to your breasts, which could result in sagging. Staying hydrated is also important to keep the skin firm. (See the chapter on nutrition and breast health.)

Exercise
You cannot firm up breast tissue with exercise because the breast tissue is not a muscle. However, underneath the breasts are muscles and connective tissues that do respond to exercise, so you can improve the appearance of your chest muscles with stretching and

weight-bearing exercises. With exercise, you must make sure that you wear an appropriate garment so that the breasts are supported and not moving unrestricted, which would place stress on the tissue.

Exercise, when done consistently and appropriately, is helpful to your overall health including your breast health. There are many exercises that you can do. Some use your own body weight and other exercises use free weights. You can join your local gym and participate in a fitness class, use a personal trainer, or exercise on your own using books or social media (e.g., YouTube videos) to find an exercise regimen that works for you. Here are a few examples of exercises you can do:

- Planks: These strengthen your overall body, including the chest.
- Push-ups: These exercise the pectoral muscles, which may help lift the breasts.
- Tricep dips: These strengthen the triceps and the pectoral muscles.
- Chest press (with dumbbells): These improve the arm and chest muscles.
- Yoga: This may stretch and strengthen the entire body and improve posture, which would improve the appearance of the breasts.

Social Habits and the Breasts

Alcohol

An alcoholic drink is one that contains the drug ethanol. It is mainly produced through fermentation of fruits or grains and is largely used for recreation. It has some health benefits and may not have a negative impact on the breasts in small quantities (e.g., one drink or less per week). But given that alcohol changes the way that estrogen is processed, it can increase the estrogen level in the breasts. If a person consumes 2-6 drinks per week or more, it has been shown to increase the risk of breast cancer.

Tobacco
Mammary tissue, like many other body parts, has the ability to hold on to the carcinogens that are found in tobacco. It is thought that some of these carcinogens may play a role in causing breast cancer. Given this information, tobacco is not good for breast health.

Marijuana
Marijuana is a plant that is sometimes used recreationally and sometimes used for medicinal reasons. It has cannabinoids, which are chemicals that help produce the effects of the nervous system that are seen with its use. It is not recommended for use while breastfeeding. More studies are needed to look at its impact on breast disease and breast cancer.

Summary Points

- The hormonal changes that occur in menopause also affect the breasts.
- Hormone replacement therapy may have an effect on the breasts. Your risk can be calculated and discussed with your health care provider.
- Breasts will sag over time.
- You can delay breast sagging with a healthy lifestyle including breast support and good posture, nutrition, and exercise.
- Social habits such as consuming alcohol and smoking may also negatively impact breast health.

CHAPTER 22

BODY IMAGE, SEXUAL HEALTH, AND YOUR BREASTS

∽❧∽

Proverbs 5:18-19 (KJV)

*Let thy fountain be blessed: and rejoice
with the wife of thy youth.*

*Let her be as the loving hind and pleasant roe;
let her breasts satisfy thee at all times; and be
thou ravished always with her love.*

Body Image

Body image is how you feel about yourself when you look in the mirror. How you feel may be different from how you look. It is all about how you think you look. Your body image is a result of many influences, including your culture, your family, your emotions, your mood, and your hormones. Not feeling good about your body image puts you at risk for risky behavior.

This point of view may be realistic (healthy) or unrealistic (unhealthy). You must decide to have a positive body image and you can also encourage others to have a positive body image. Always love yourself and accept your body. Keep in mind the positive things about your body and pay attention to your own biases and beliefs about your body, including your breasts.

1 Corinthians 6:19-20 (ESV)

Or do you not know that your body is a
temple of the Holy Spirit within you, whom
you have from God? You are not your own, for you
were bought with a price. So glorify God in your body.

Psalm 139:14 (ESV)

I praise you, for I am fearfully and wonderfully made.
Wonderful are your works; my soul knows it very well.

Sexual Health

Sexual health as defined by the World Health Organization as "… a state of physical, emotional, mental and social well-being in relation to sexuality; it is not merely the absence of disease, dysfunction or infirmity. Sexual health requires a positive and respectful approach to sexuality and sexual relationships, as well as the possibility of having pleasurable and safe sexual experiences, free of coercion, discrimination and violence. For sexual health to be attained and maintained, the sexual rights of all persons must be respected, protected and fulfilled." (WHO, 2006). In other words, sexual health is defined as the well-being of your physical, social, and mental health as is relates to your sexual function.

Every woman's sexual experience is unique to them. Having an open and positive attitude can only help your sexual experience. The breasts play a role in this experience. There are three sensory maps in the brain—specifically in the parietal cortex which lights up in functional MRI images when the genitals are stimulated. One represents the clitoris, another the vagina, and the third represents the cervix. These maps also receive input when the nipples are stimulated. From a functional perspective, this means that the breasts doubles as a sexual organ and can be a source of sexual pleasure for many women.

The sexual response cycle is divided into three phases: desire, arousal, and orgasm. Each stage is associated with different physiological changes. The breasts also respond and change with each phase of this cycle. Short-term changes affect your breast size during and after sex. For example, sex temporarily changes the shape and appearance of your breasts due to changes in blood circulation. As a result, the breasts look and feel fuller and they may appear more upright. The skin also looks different—the areola will tighten when the muscles behind the breasts contract. The nipples become erect when they are stimulated and are therefore more noticeable during sex.

Table 15

Physical Changes in Breasts During Sexual Response	
Desire	No specific changes.
Arousal	Nipples become erect and/or darker in color. Breast size increases.
Orgasm	Breast size may increase more as they become more engorged. Changes that came with arousal may persist.
Resolution	Nipples and breasts return to their normal size and color.

If you are postpartum or breastfeeding, you may find that your breasts leak when you are sexually aroused or if you orgasm.

Currently, there is no scientific evidence that frequent sexual activity has any permanent effect on the breasts.

Factors such as medications, age, relationship with a partner, and psychiatric and medical disorders may affect a lady's ability to respond to sexual contact. Counseling to overcome stigma and enhance awareness on sexuality is an essential step in management.

1 Corinthians 6:19-20 (ESV)
Or do you not know that your body is a temple of
the Holy Spirit within you, whom you have from
God? You are not your own, for you were bought
with a price. So, glorify God in your body.

Summary Points

- Body image describes how you view your body, including your breasts.
- Healthy body image is important.
- Breasts play a part in sexual health.
- The breasts change temporarily during sex.
- Breasts may be a source of orgasm for some.

CHAPTER 23
VITAMINS, HERBAL SUPPLEMENTS, AND BREAST CARE

Genesis 1:29-30 (KJV)

And God said, Behold, I have given you every herb bearing seed, which is upon the face of all the earth, and every tree, in which is the fruit of a tree yielding seed; to you it shall be for meat.

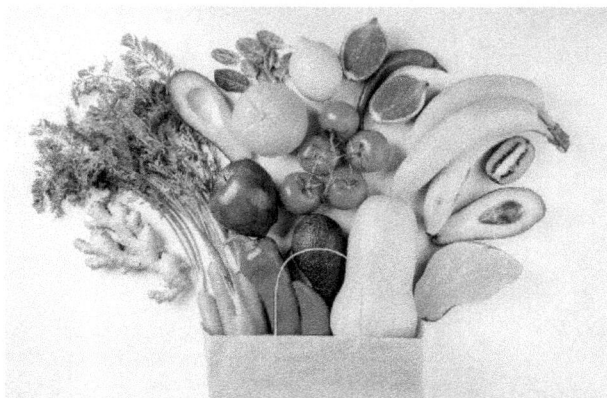

Figure 41 A grocery bag with food items beneficial to breast health

We often say, "You are what you eat." No one can dispute the importance of diet in your overall health. The food that you eat forms the building blocks for your body and the fuel for the functions that your body carries out on a daily basis.

The idea behind supplements and herbs is that they contain substances or compounds that are helpful to the way our cells grow and function. The following information should be reviewed with your health care providers. These foods are meant to provide sources of antioxidants or substances that are useful in killing bad cells in the body.

Meat eaters have an increased risk of breast cancer compared to non-meat eaters. Chemical additives, hormones, and natural additives such as sugar, salt, and flour are used to help preserve foods, but they are also responsible for causing damage to cells in the body, including in the breasts.

Pay attention not only to what you are eating, but to how the food is prepared. The cooking methods that we tend to like the best are the ones that may not be as good for us (because of the changes that occur during the cooking process). For example, when you grill foods, carcinogens are formed on the food's skin. When you fry foods cancer causing substances are formed in the food, as acrylamide.

Food For Breast Cancer Prevention

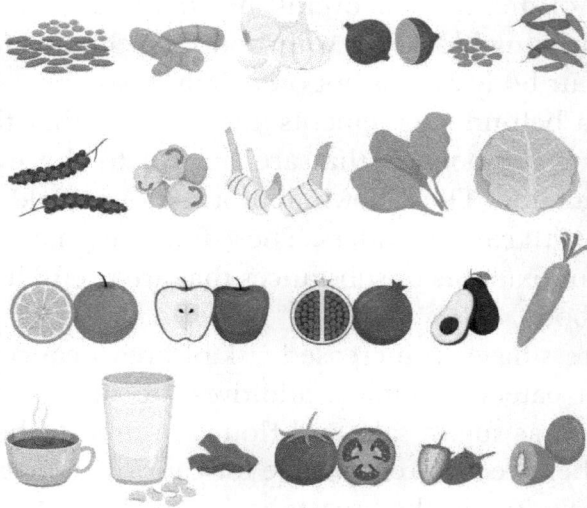

Figure 42 Fruits, vegetables, and supplements that help to maintain breast health

Foods for Breast Health

Lentils
Lentils (Lens culinaris), dried beans, and split peas contain folate, thiamin (Vitamin B1) and antioxidants. They have been shown to decrease the risk of benign breast diseases as well as breast cancer.

Turmeric
Turmeric is a spice that comes from the turmeric plant. It has a component in it called curcumin which has an anti-inflammatory and anticancer effect. Turmeric may interfere with chemotherapy for breast cancer so avoid it if you are undergoing treatment.

Onion and Garlic
Garlic, known by its scientific name allium sativum, has a high sulfur content. It also contains other beneficial components such

as arginine, oligosaccharides, flavonoids, and selenium. The components in garlic can activate the enzymes that break down chemical cancer agents and cause cells to die when they are supposed to (apoptosis). They can also help stop cancer cell growth (proliferation) and cut down on the movement and penetration of abnormal cells. Garlic has been shown to decrease DNA strand breaks induced by carcinogens. Garlic also affects the genetic material in abnormal cells, causing them to stop growing. As a result, studies have shown that high consumption of onions, garlic, and leeks were associated with lower risk of breast cancer.

Almonds, Peanuts or Walnuts
Researchers found that eating seeds, nuts and legumes, which includes beans, lentils, soybeans, and corn, may all reduce the risk of benign breast conditions (and therefore, breast cancer).

Peppers
Red peppers have both capsaicin and antioxidant carotenoids. They contain a cancer-fighting compound called curcumin which can inhibit many types of cancer cells, including breast.

Green peppers are rich in chlorophyll which can bind cancer-causing carcinogens in certain body parts.

Grapes
Grapes are a good source of flavonols, phenolic acids, resveratrol, flavan-3-ols, tannins (proanthocyanidins and ellagitannins) and anthocyanins (in red and purple grapes). They are thought to help prevent DNA damage and may help prevent the growth of abnormal cells. The components in grapes are good for helping regulate and maintain overall breast health.

Mushrooms
Some types of mushrooms reduce the growth of cancer cells. They also stop aromatase (an enzyme that plays a role in the production

of estrogen). Mushrooms are rich in polysaccharides and beta-glu-
cans which are active in enhancing the immune system. They are
also good sources of niacin (Vitamin B3) and riboflavin (Vitamin
B2). Mushroom types that have been studied and shown to be beneficial include:

- White button mushrooms (Agaaricus bisporous)
- Shitake mushrooms (Lentinus edodes)
- Maitake mushrooms (Grifola frondosa)

Ginger
Ginger has a property known as selective cytotoxicity. It stops the
proliferation of breast cancer cells without affecting normal breast
cells. This property is very beneficial for breast health.

Kale
Kale contains significant levels of Vitamins C and K and is a great
source of beta-Carotene, lutein, and other components which have
been reported to help cells die when they should (apoptosis). Kale
has also been shown to help prevent the abnormal formation of
blood vessels and is thought to decrease the biproducts of estrogen
break down, thereby promoting breast health.

Cabbage
Cabbage is a leafy vegetable that comes in several colors including green, red, and purple. It is a cruciferous vegetable and is related to broccoli, brussels sprouts, and cauliflower. Cabbage has
the highest levels of two anticancer glucosinolates out of all of the
cruciferous vegetables. These glucosinolates help trigger enzyme
defenses and may inhibit tumor growth. The protective effects
of cabbage work best when it is either blanched or eaten raw (as
in sauerkraut) since it loses its potency with heating. Cabbage is
packed with nutrients and it's recommended that you consume

it several times a week. One cup of green cabbage only has 20 calories yet provides 102% of your daily Vitamin K intake and 45% of your daily Vitamin C intake.

Citrus
Citrus fruits have limonoids which are anti-inflammatory and anti-proliferative (meaning they decrease cell growth). Citrus is helpful in maintaining breast health.

Seaweed
The category of seaweed, or ocean vegetables, includes edible seaweed or algae such as dulse, kelp nori, and sea lettuce. Seaweed is a good dietary source of many minerals such as calcium manganese, magnesium, and many vitamins including Vitamins A, B12, C, E, and K. Seaweed has been shown to have anti-inflammatory, antioxidant, anticoagulant, and antibiotic properties which are all beneficial to breast health.

Tomatoes
Tomatoes are good sources of carotenoids, lycopene, and melatonin. They can help lower inflammation, decrease estrogen production, and aid in cell repair. They are beneficial for breast health.

Apples
Apples are packed with fiber (pectin), Vitamin C, and carotenoids. They have been shown to decrease your risk of cancers including breast cancer.

Pomegranate
These fruits have substances that are thought to help prevent breast cancer. Pomegranates have certain phytochemicals that are called ellagitannins which are shown to inhibit the growth of estrogen-responsive breast cancer. It is also thought that they

can help prevent and decrease cancer through lowering inflammation and encouraging the death of cells that are abnormal.

Avocado
Avocado is a good source of fiber, Vitamin B6, folate, and lutein (a carotenoid). They are also a good source of monounsaturated fats and rich in cytochrome P-450s, which are enzymes involved in drug metabolism and estrogen metabolism. These substances are thought to be helpful in maintaining breast health.

Carrots
Carrots are a root vegetable that come in many colors. They contain carotene, fiber, Vitamin K1, potassium, antioxidants, fiber, minerals, and other phytochemicals, which may be beneficial for breast health. The possible relationship between carrot intake and breast cancer risk has been looked into in epidemiological studies. However, the results were not consistent, with some studies finding a significant inverse association, while others did not.

Strawberries
Strawberries are thought to have substances that support breast health such as ellagic acid and ellagitannins, Vitamin B9, Vitamin C, and others.

Kiwi
Kiwi contains ursolic acid and substances that have been shown to help with repairing DNA breakage and enhancing the immune system.

Green Tea
Green tea contains polyphenols. These are thought to be helpful in reducing cell damage, which may sometimes lead to cancer in the body. Green tea may help to maintain breast health.

Soy

Soy is recommended in moderation. The isoflavones (plant estrogens) that are found in soy have some benefits. Animal studies have shown an increase in risk of breast cancer when consumed in high amounts, but human studies show different results. It is important to discuss the use of these products with your health care provider.

Fatty Acids

Dietary fats may be modifiers of breast cancer risk. Specific polyunsaturated fats such as Omega-3 polyunsaturated fats are thought to have anticancer effects. These can be found in foods such as flaxseed, soybeans, and fish.

Supplements and Breast Health

Cat's claw

This is called Uncaria and is found in South America. It comes in two species: Uncaria guianensis and Uncaria tomentosa. It has immune stimulant and antioxidant properties that are being studied in breast cancer patients. It is made up of components that can theoretically kill and stop the growth of cells. Additional studies are needed on this extract.

Vitamin E

Vitamin E is an antioxidant that may help decrease pain and inflammation and may lower your risk of breast cancer. You can try taking 1200 mg per day.

Evening Primrose Oil

Evening primrose oil is made from the seeds of a North American plant. It contains gamma linolenic acid which is an Omega-6 fatty acid that is thought to decrease inflammation and pain. You may try taking 1-3 grams or 2.4 ml per day for 6 months.

Flax Seeds

Flax seeds (linum usitatissimum) have phytoestrogen lignans. These are changed as they are broken down in the colon. This conversion in the gut helps the anticancer effects of the flax seeds. It also helps block inflammatory agents such as interleukin 1 (IL-1). A study out of Canada noted that flax seeds are linked to the prevention of breast cancer. Flax seed oil is also known to reduce breast cancer growth. Flax seeds are a good source of vitamins and minerals such as Vitamin B1, selenium, manganese, magnesium, phosphorous, and zinc. However, flax seed intake has to be monitored as it can cause bleeding issues and problems with the bowels. Only a small daily serving of flax seeds is required to improve breast health. Try 1-4 teaspoons of ground flax seeds per day.

Vitamin D

Vitamin D reduces the risk of cancers including breast cancer. However, we have yet to determine the optimal dose. Your health care provider may recommend that you check your Vitamin D levels. Vitamin D can be found in fortified milk, fortified foods, and exposure to sunlight.

Vitamin B Complex

Some studies have shown a decrease in breast cancer risk with thiamine and pyridoxine intake, but no other decrease in breast cancer risk has been noted in other studies. Folate may be beneficial in non- to low-alcohol drinkers.

Summary Points

- Many foods provide vitamins and mineral that may be helpful in the prevention of breast cancer or maintaining overall breast health.
- As research continues, we will find out what things are helpful and harmful in breast cancer and maintaining breast health.

APPENDIX A

⁓⦸⁓

Common Questions About Breast Health

How often should I have my breasts checked? You should consider checking your own breasts once a month and having your breasts checked by a health care provider once a year.

When is the best time of the month to examine my breasts? The best time of the month to examine the breasts is one week after your menstrual cycle.

Should I consider genetic testing for breast cancer? Discuss this with your health care provider. If they think you are at increased risk for developing breast cancer, they will recommend that you proceed with genetic testing.

Can you achieve an orgasm by stimulation of your breasts? Yes, your breasts have nerve endings and this is possible.

I have my family to take care of, how can I take the time for me? If you are not well, you cannot take care of your family. Make a schedule and put time for yourself in it. Carve out some time to take care or your concerns.

Can I breastfeed if I have breast cancer? Yes. Cancer cells are not transferred into breast milk; therefore, breastfeeding is safe. An exception to this is if you are receiving chemotherapy or a drug called tamoxifen, as these drugs can pass into breast milk and are harmful to the nursing infant. If you recently had breast surgery, it may be best not to breastfeed. The surgeon who performed your surgery will advise you appropriately.

The tumor or surgery on the breasts can affect the system of tubes (ducts) that carry and produce breast milk, resulting in a decrease in milk. If you notice your breast milk supply is low, you will have to supplement feeding with infant formula. You can consult with your oncologist, obstetrician, and pediatrician to come up with a solution that works best for you.

Does sex cause your breasts to sag? No, it does not. Sagging of the breasts (ptosis) is most likely a result of smoking, weight loss, or aging.

Are breastfeeding and bottle feeding the same? No, they are not. Breastfeeding has many benefits for the baby and the mother (see chapter on breastfeeding).

How does estrogen affect the breasts? In early puberty when there is less estrogen, the breast tissue is denser. As menstruation starts, the estrogen levels change, and the breasts change in response. In menopause, the estrogen level drops and the tissue in the breasts changes as it becomes fattier.

What do I do if I have a family history of breast cancer? You should discuss this with your physician. They will decide if genetic testing would be helpful in your case. They would also make a decision about when you should start to have imaging and what type of imaging would be best. They will also make additional recommendations to help reduce your risk of cancer.

I had a mammogram last year and it was normal. Do I have to do one this year? A mammogram is a screening test that will show any abnormalities that are present at the time that you are imaged. But that imaging may change with time. Follow the recommendation and guidelines of your health care provider.

Can you use supplements for breast enlargement? Some supplements are purported to increase the size of the breasts, but there is no literature to support this.

How long can I breastfeed my baby? You can breastfeed for six months to two years.

I saw some blood in my breast milk, is that normal? Blood may be a normal finding if it is caused by blood vessels that break when you are breastfeeding. It can also be caused by cracked nipples or an infection. Since there are normal and abnormal causes of blood in the breast milk, you should discuss this with your health care provider.

I am breastfeeding and pregnant. Should I stop breastfeeding? It is safe to breastfeed while pregnant, but you should be aware that some ladies will have contractions while breastfeeding.

One of my breasts is bigger than the other, should I be worried? It is normal to have some difference in size between each breast. Sometimes the difference can be 10-25%. If you are concerned, discuss this with your health care professional who can tell you if the size difference is normal and provide treatment options if indicated.

Why do I have pain on and off in my breast? People have breast pain for many reasons. It is important to discuss this with your health care provider. You can keep a record of when it happens, on which side, and what makes it better or worse. This may help your health care provider figure out why you are having pain.

APPENDIX B

❧

Exercises to Improve Appearance of the Breasts

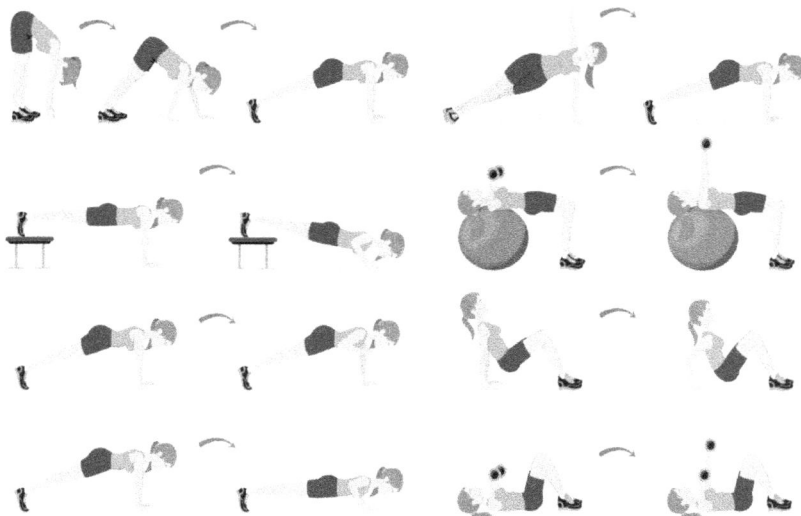

CHEST WORKOUT

Arm And Back Workout

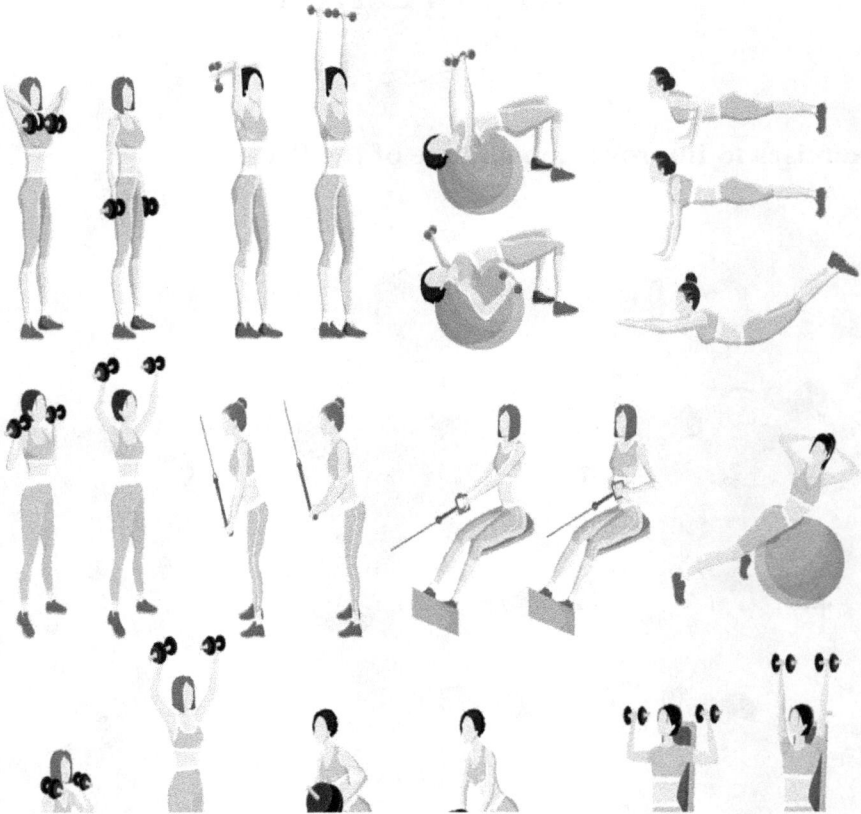

Exercises to strengthen back muscles and abdomen

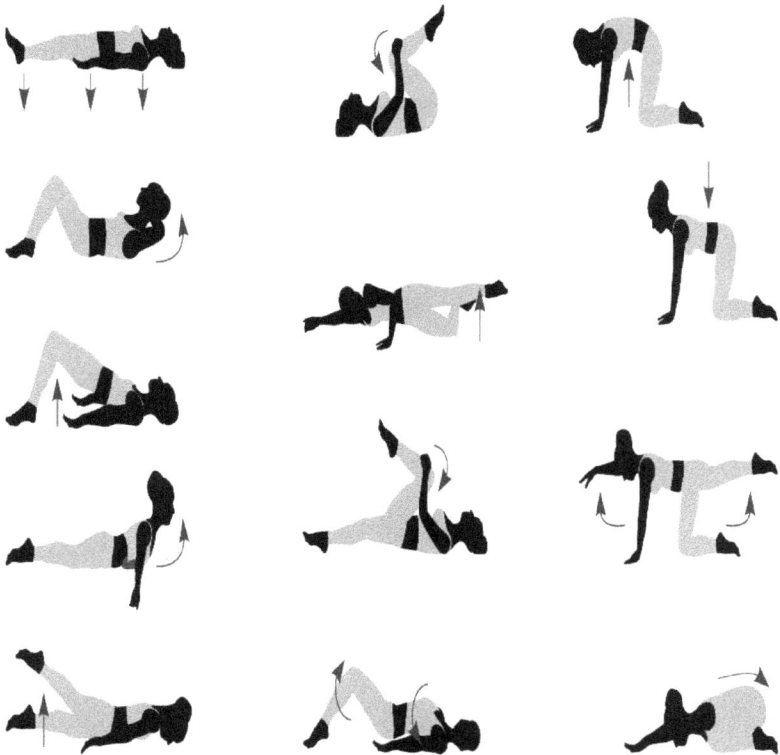

Pages for your thoughts and questions

INDEX

Page numbers followed by "*f*" and "*t*" refer to figures and tables respectively.

B

BCS. *See* Breast conserving
surgery (BCS)
Bell shaped breasts, 23
Benign lesions. *See* Lesions
BGSI. *See* Breast-specific gamma
imaging (BGSI)
BIA-ALCL. *See* Breast-implant
associated-anaplastic large
cell lymphoma (BIA-ALCL)
Biopsy, 141–143
core, 142
large core, 142
sentinel lymph node, 145
stereotactic core, 142
ultrasound-guided, 141, 141*f*
vacuum-assisted, 142–143
BI-RADS. *See* Breast Imaging
Reporting and Database
System Scoring (BI-RADS)
Birth control pills, 112, 181–182
Blocked duct, breastfeeding, 168
Blood supply, 19–21
Bloodwork, 11
Body image, 192–193
Botfly, 79
Bras, 36–39
anatomy of, 40*f*
determining size, 37–39, 38*f*
BRCA genes, 113–114, 113*f*
BRCA 1, 114
BRCA 2, 114
Breast(s)

anatomy, 15*f*, 16–19, 17*f*,
18*f*, 19*f*
appearance, 21–25, 22*f*
blood supply, 19–21
development, 14–16, 15*t*
inspection, 10
menstrual cycle and, 26–29, 28*f*
physical examination, 10
regions/quadrants, 16–17, 16*f*
Breast cancer, 117–138
adenocarcinoma, 120–121
adenoid cystic carcinoma
(ACC), 124–125
angiosarcoma, 124
BIA-ALCL, 125
defined, 118
HER2-enriched, 127
inflammatory, 123
lobular neoplasia, 122–123
luminal A, 127
luminal B, 127
lymphoma, 125
metastasis, 125
normal-like, 128
Paget's disease of nipple,
123–124
plasmacytoma, 126
receptors, 126
removal of lesion, 128
risk factors, 109–115
staging, 130–136, 136*f*
subtypes, 126–128
symptoms, 118

I

Imaging, 11, 41–53
  alternative screenings methods, 52–53
  defined, 41
  electrical impedance imaging, 52
  indication for, 42
  mammography, 43–49
  MBI, 50
  MRI, 50–51
  optical imaging tests, 52
  PET, 51
  PET-CT scan, 51
  PET-MRI scan, 52
  thermography, 52
  ultrasound, 49
  ultrasound elastography, 53
Immunomodulators for breast cancer, 130
Immunotherapy for breast cancer, 129
Infections, 73–81
  abscesses, 76
  actinomyces, 77
  cysticercosis, 79
  filariasis, 78
  granulomatous mastitis, 77
  inflammation, 73
  lupus mastitis, 80–81
  mammary duct ectasia, 74
  mastitis, 76
  Mondor's disease, 74–75

  myiasis, 79
  schistosomiasis, 79–80
  tuberculosis, 76–77
  worm and parasitic, 78–80
  yeast, 80
Infiltrating syringomatous adenoma, 71–72
Inflammation, 73. *See also* Mastitis
Inflammatory breast cancer, 123
Inspection of breasts, 10
Internal medicine doctors, 5
Intertrigo, 94–95
Intraductal papilloma, 91–92

J

Juvenile breast hypertrophy, 103

K

Kale, 200
Kiwi, 202

L

Large core biopsy, 142
Lentils, 198
Lesions, 62–72
  adenoma, 64–65
  causes of, 64
  cysts, 66–67
  epidermal inclusion cyst, 67
  fat necrosis, 69
  fibrocystic changes, 66
  fibroepithelial, 65–66
  galactocele, 68

Periductal mastitis. *See* Mammary duct ectasia

Personal history, as risk factors for breast cancer, 111

PET. *See* Positron emission tomography (PET)

Phyllodes tumor, 65–66

Physical examination, 9–10

Physician's assistants, 4

Plasmacytoma, 126

Plastic surgery, 146–158
anesthesia, 155
complications, 153–155
costs, 157–158
defined, 147
non-surgical procedures, 148–149
post surgery instruction list, 155–156
satisfaction, 156–157
selecting surgeon, 147–148
surgical procedures, 149–153

PMDD. *See* Premenstrual dysphoric disorder (PMDD)

PMS. *See* Premenstrual syndrome (PMS)

Polyarteritis nodosa, 104

Polymastia, 58

Polythelia, 58

Pomegranate, 201–202

Positions for breastfeeding, 166, 166*f*

Positron emission tomography (PET), 51

Positron emission tomography-CT (PET-CT) scan, 51

Positron emission tomography-MRI (PET-MRI) scan, 52

Prayer, 137

Pregnancy, breast changes with, 162

Premenstrual dysphoric disorder (PMDD), 84

Premenstrual syndrome (PMS), 84

Primary hypothyroidism, 91

Pseudoangiomatous stromal hyperplasia (PASH), 102

Psoriasis, 99

Puberty, 14

Purulent discharge, 88. *See also* Nipple discharge

R

Radiation exposure
breast cancer, 129
mammography and, 47–48, 48*t*

Relaxed breasts, 23

Removal of lesion, 128

Rheumatologists, 5

Risk assessment, 114–115

Risk factors for breast cancer, 109–115
age, 110
breast density, 111
exposure to radiation, 112–113
family history, 111
gender, 110

selection of, 147–148
Surgery, nipple discharge and, 91
Surgical procedures, plastic
    surgery, 149–153
Suspensory ligaments, 18

T

Targeted antibodies for breast
    cancer, 129
Teardrop breasts, 24
Testosterone, 187
Therapeutic breast procedures,
    140, 143–145
Thermography, 52
3D mammogram tomosynthesis,
    49
3D mammography, 43
Tietze syndrome, 85–86
Tinea versicolor, 97–98
TM. *See* Total mastectomy (TM)
Tobacco, 191
Tomatoes, 201
Total mastectomy (TM), 144
Transitional milk, 164
Trauma, nipple discharge and,
    91
Triple-negative/basal-like breast
    cancer, 127
Tuberculosis, 76–77
Tubular breasts, 60
Tumbu fly, 79
Tumors, 130, 131–132
    nipple, 71–72

Tumor suppressor genes, 113–114,
    113*f*
Turmeric, 198

U

Ultrasound, 49
    sarcoidosis, 102
Ultrasound elastography, 53
Ultrasound-guided biopsy, 141, 141*f*
Underproduction of milk, 170
US Preventative Task Force, 42

V

Vacuum-assisted biopsy, 142–143
Vascular disease, 103
Vitamin B complex, 204
Vitamin D, 204
Vitamin E, 203

W

Walnuts, 199
Wegner's disease. *See*
    Granulomatosis with
    polyangiitis (GPA)
World Health Organization, 193
Worm and parasitic, 78–80
Wuchereria bancrofti, 78

X

X-ray mammography, 44–45, 45*f*

Y

Yeast infections, 80

www.ingramcontent.com/pod-product-compliance
Lightning Source LLC
Chambersburg PA
CBHW031506270326
41930CB00006B/270